With love to my husband, Dave Foster; son, Alan; and daughter, Melissa; for all their support and patience, and my parents, John and Toby McDonell, who always said ''You can do it.'' And thanks to my special and creative friend Kathy Zell for listening and sharing.

E.F.

To my husband, Dennis Hartinger, who put in double duty to free up my time and provided the support whenever I needed someone to listen; my children, Christopher, Joshua, Travis, and Nicole for their understanding and patience; and my dear friends Lorraine and Joe Buckstein for their caring and support.

K.H.

To my mother and father, Shirley and William Smith; my sister, Kimberley; and my brothers, Christopher and Anthony. I thank them for their love, support, and encouragement. I would also like to thank Dr. Jim Rog and Dr. Glen Reif of The University of Maine. Their energy and enthusiasm for physical education motivated me to further my education. Finally, I would like to thank my friend Laird McLennan, who taught me that what young people need most is a friend.

K.S.

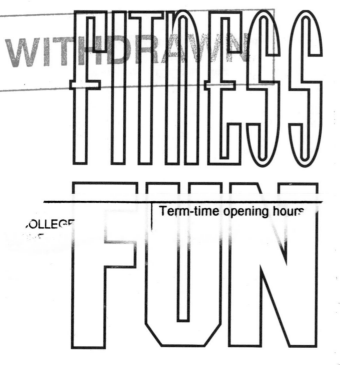

FITNESS

Term-time opening hours

,OLLEGE

FUN

2005

Emily R. Foster, MAT
Sabin Early Childhood Education Center
Portland, Oregon

Karyn Hartinger, MS
Butter Creek School
Aloha, Oregon

Katherine A. Smith, MS
Madawaska Elementary Schools
Madawaska, Maine

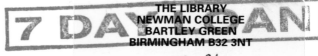

Human Kinetics

Library of Congress Cataloging-in-Publication Data

Foster, Emily R., 1947-
   Fitness fun / Emily R. Foster, Karyn Hartinger, Katherine A.
Smith.
     p.   cm.
   ISBN 0-87322-384-5
   1. Physical education for children--United States. 2. Physical
fitness for children--United States.   I. Hartinger, Karyn, 1951-
. II. Smith, Katherine A., 1961-   . III. Title.
   GV223.F67   1992
   372.86--dc20   92-10626
                                                       CIP

ISBN: 0-87322-384-5

Acquisitions Editor: Rick Frey, PhD; Developmental Editor: Larret Galasyn-Wright; Assistant Editors: Elizabeth Bridgett, Valerie Hall, and Moyra Knight; Copyeditor: Dianna Matlosz; Proofreader: Dawn Barker; Production Director: Ernie Noa; Typesetter: Angela K. Snyder; Text Design: Keith Blomberg; Text Layout: Denise Peters and Angela K. Snyder; Cover Design: Jack Davis; Illustrations: Mary Yemma Long; Printer: United Graphics

Human Kinetics books are available at special discounts for bulk purchase. Special editions or book excerpts can also be created to specification. For details, contact the Special Sales Manager at Human Kinetics.

Printed in the United States of America   10 9 8 7 6 5

Human Kinetics
P.O. Box 5076, Champaign, IL 61825-5076
1-800-747-4457

Canada: Human Kinetics, Box 24040, Windsor, ON N8Y 4Y9
1-800-465-7301 (in Canada only)

Europe: Human Kinetics, P.O. Box IW14, Leeds LS16 6TR, United Kingdom
(44) 1132 781708

Australia: Human Kinetics, 2 Ingrid Street, Clapham 5062, South Australia
(08) 371 3755

New Zealand: Human Kinetics, P.O. Box 105-231, Auckland 1
(09) 523 3462

Contents

About the Authors   vii
Preface   ix

Introduction   **1**

Cardiorespiratory Fitness   1
Muscular Strength   3
Muscular Endurance   4
Flexibility   4
FIT   4

Teaching Tips   **7**

Management   7
Age Appropriateness   8
Equipment   8
Safety   9

How to Use This Book   **11**

Understanding the Fitness Symbols   11
Using the Game Finder   12

Game Finder   **13**

Part I   Warm-Up Activities   *19*
Part II   Quick Activities   *41*
Part III   Main Activities   *73*

About the Authors

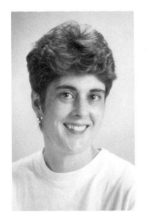 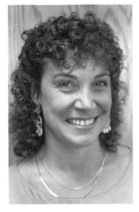 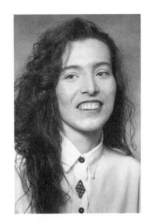

Emily Foster   Karyn Hartinger   Katherine Smith

Emily Foster, MAT, is an elementary physical education specialist for the Portland Public Schools in Oregon. She received her master's degree in teaching physical education from Lewis and Clark College in 1981, and has been teaching and creating new activities ever since. She has also written physical education and fitness curricula for the Portland school district. Ms. Foster is a member of the American Alliance for Health, Physical Education, Recreation and Dance (AAHPERD), the Oregon Alliance for Health, Physical Education, Recreation and Dance (OAHPERD), the National Association for Sports and Physical Education (NASPE), and the Northwest Council for Children's Expanded Physical Education (NCCEPE).

Karyn Hartinger, MS, is a physical education specialist for the Reedville School District in Aloha, Oregon. In 1982 she received her master's degree in physical education from Portland State University. Ms. Hartinger has been voted Oregon's Physical Education Teacher of the Year for the elementary level and has been a member of the Portland School District Curriculum Committee. She is a member of AAHPERD, OAHPERD, NASPE, and NCCEPE.

Katherine A. Smith, MS, is a health, fitness, and physical education specialist in Madawaska, Maine. She received her masters degree in physical education from Montana State University in 1985, and has since written curricula for health and physical education for school districts in Maine, Colorado, Montana, and Oregon. Ms. Smith is a member of AAHPERD, NASPE, and the Maine Alliance for Health, Physical Education, Recreation and Dance.

Preface

Recently, there has been an increased concern regarding the fitness level of children. The lifestyles of today's young people include television, computer games, and fast food. Hours formerly spent playing out-of-doors with neighborhood friends are being spent at more sedentary activities. This change in lifestyle has produced a nation of unfit children who are unaware of their poor fitness. They do not realize the necessity of maintaining a healthy body, and they lack the knowledge of how to improve.

As educators, we have the opportunity to initiate healthful changes in young people that will enrich their lives! To do this, we must motivate children to care for themselves and their own well-being. We must help them become excited about fitness by showing them that becoming fit means learning new and exciting concepts and that exercising really can be fun and rewarding!

Fitness Fun is designed to help you meet the fitness education challenge. Whether you are a seasoned physical educator or a recent graduate just beginning a career as a physical education specialist, you will benefit from the material offered here. Classroom teachers, program directors, recreation specialists, and coaches also will find exciting and useful ideas in this book. Our learning activities have specific fitness goals and each page is easy to read and understand so you can review activities quickly and put them into use immediately!

Fitness Fun provides 85 exciting and innovative activities to help you develop cardiorespiratory fitness, muscular strength, muscular endurance, and flexibility in young people. Warm-ups, quick activities, and main activities make up the three sections of this book.

All of the activities in *Fitness Fun* are field-tested fitness enhancers. The games are success-oriented, and most utilize individual equipment. Waiting lines have been eliminated. Children at a variety of fitness levels can participate together in these activities and still enjoy personal success.

Fitness Fun offers several activities that require children to compete with themselves. They allow students to improve their own fitness levels and to accomplish tasks at their own pace. Group and partner activities challenge students to work together to perform specific tasks. Competitive games are included in *Fitness Fun*, too. Lessons with a variety of individually challenging activities, mixed with group activities and competitive games from time to time, will motivate all students.

The key to getting children involved in their own personal fitness is *fun*! When young people are offered exciting learning experiences they discover the pleasures of moving and playing for fitness enhancement. And the interest in these activities that children develop today can influence their behavior all their lives.

We know you will find the games and activities in *Fitness Fun* useful as you strive to develop fitness and a healthier lifestyle in the young people you work with.

Introduction

Children need to be aware of the importance of being physically active and know how to take responsibility for their own fitness. If children are taught the benefits of exercise they can better understand that exercise and fitness are an avenue to a better quality of life. Children need to know the consequences of a sedentary lifestyle void of physical activity and that high blood pressure and cholesterol levels, shortness of breath, and fatigue are all factors that they can control through exercise.

Fitness Fun is designed to provide children with unique activities they look forward to doing. The traditional (but usually unmotivating) regimen of sit-ups, push-ups, and laps can be replaced with games, activities, and variations that motivate and interest all of the participants. Instructors who show interest and enthusiasm and believe in what they are teaching will motivate students as the children see that they are truly concerned about student progress.

We want children to become fit while still accommodating individual differences. Your students have different levels of fitness, and you cannot expect them all to perform the same way. They should be allowed to pace themselves and adjust the intensity of activities to suit their own fitness levels. The games we've provided let children make these decisions.

Use a variety of games, activities, and exercise variations to keep your students interested. Providing different learning activities will keep students excited about exercise and eager to know what they will do next!

You should address four basic components in teaching children about fitness: cardiorespiratory fitness, muscular strength, muscular endurance, and flexibility. Children need to do activities to develop each of these areas.

Cardiorespiratory Fitness

Cardiorespiratory fitness is the efficient functioning of body systems, particularly heart, lungs, and blood vessels, during and after exercise. As the cardiovascular system becomes more efficient, the body can work harder for longer periods. The heart becomes stronger, and the lungs and blood vessels can better deliver oxygen throughout the body. Children will become stronger and more energetic by following a regular cardiorespiratory fitness program. They will discover that they can work and play for longer periods without getting tired.

Talk-Jog Rule: Initially, you must present low-intensity, short-duration aerobic activities. Children can exercise more vigorously as their fitness levels improve. Stress the "talk-jog" rule; children should work at a level that allows them to talk comfortably with a friend while exercising.

Heart Rate: Another way children can monitor their exercise intensity is by keeping track of their heart rates. Checking their pulses from time to time will tell them if they are working too hard or not hard enough. The easiest place for a child to locate the pulse is at the neck or wrist.

To find the carotid artery on the neck, students should place two fingers side by side on the "Adam's apple," then slide them into the groove on either side of the neck. Children should be able to feel a pulse. If they cannot, have them slowly move their fingers up or down until they find the heartbeat. Remind them to press gently.

To locate a pulse on the radial artery of the wrist, children should hold one hand, palm up, and place two fingers of the other hand side by side approximately 1 inch from the wrist on the thumb side. Students should not use the thumb to locate the pulse because it also has a pulse. You may have to help some children locate their pulses when their fingers are in place. Tell the children to tap on their thighs each time they feel a beat so you can observe them practicing.

To use a visual method of counting the heartbeat, take a toothpick, stick it into a ball of clay the size of a pea, and place the clay on the radial artery. The toothpick will move back and forth with every heartbeat. Have students hold their arms steady by lying on the floor.

Target Heart Rate: The target heart rate is a range in which students should exercise to improve cardiorespiratory fitness. This determines the appropriate intensity level for each student's workout. Use the following formula to calculate a target heart rate for each of your students.

220			220	
−( )	Age		−( )	Age
=( )	Maximum heart rate		=( )	Maximum heart rate
−( )	Resting heart rate		−( )	Resting heart rate
=( ) × .65			=( ) × .85	

=( )			=( )	
+( )	Resting heart rate		+( )	Resting heart rate
=( )	Low end of the target pulse range		=( )	High end of the target pulse range

Muscular Strength

Muscular strength is the force a muscle exerts against a resistance. Children need muscular strength to meet the daily demands placed upon their bodies. Having sufficient muscular strength enables them to maintain good posture, to push and pull objects, and to enhance performance in games and sports. When you challenge students to perform tasks that require strength, you demonstrate the importance of conditioning.

Overload: Children must place an overload on the muscles they want to strengthen. To do this, they must, on a regular basis, work harder than normal. A student who wants to improve upper body strength must do exercises such as a seal-walk, crabwalk, push-ups, and pull-ups. These will tax the muscles of the upper body.

Progressive Training: Present strength training exercises *progressively* by slowly increasing the difficulty of an exercise. For example, if you want children to be able to do standard push-ups with their hands and toes on the floor, start them on variations of push-ups, such as standing push-ups against a wall or handwalking to a line on the floor while supporting their body weight on their hands. You want children to be challenged, but you do not want to overwhelm them with unrealistic expectations. This only discourages them.

Practical Training: Always try to relate to their own lives the experiences you are giving children. Provide examples so they understand how they use strength from day to day. Ask students to do a pull-up; then ask them if they could pull themselves up onto a window sill to get out of danger. Or have them remember a time when they tried to lift a heavy box. Presenting examples of practical applications of muscular strength will help students understand why muscular strength is important.

Muscular Endurance

Muscular endurance is a muscle's ability to contract and relax over an extended period without tiring. Children move constantly requiring their muscles to work for long periods. With good muscular endurance, children can participate in activities such as aerobic dance, roller skating, walking, jogging, cross-country skiing, and swimming.

Suppose your students need to improve their running endurance. Have them visualize the muscles that they use in a soccer game. "Seeing" their leg muscles work will help them better understand why they need to work their legs during conditioning. Children participate with much more desire and enthusiasm when they understand the purpose and benefits of an activity.

Flexibility

Flexibility is the range of motion of a joint and its surrounding muscles. The greater the range of motion, the more the muscles, tendons, and ligaments surrounding the joint can bend or flex. Flexibility is necessary for performing everyday activities, preventing injury, and maintaining general health. Young people often underestimate the value of stretching before and after physical activity. Help them make a habit of stretching in order to ready their bodies for activity and to prevent injuries and muscle soreness.

Static Stretching: Flexibility is maintained and increased by performing movement patterns that slowly and progressively stretch a muscle beyond its normal length at rest. Teach children to stretch their muscles statically. This means to stretch a muscle slowly and steadily without forcing or bouncing, then holding the stretch for 10 to 15 seconds.

Design the stretching portion of the session to stretch the primary muscles that will be used for the physical activity. Your students should never feel pain while performing the exercises. Tell them to stretch until they feel a "slight tug" and then hold the stretch at that point.

FIT

Teach the FIT principle. F stands for *frequency*, the number of times each week they should exercise; I is the *intensity* of the exercise; and

T stands for the *time* or duration of each exercise session. Sessions should last at least 30 minutes, 3 to 5 times a week, and incorporate all four fitness components. Children need to understand the FIT principle so they can plan exercise programs that will improve or maintain their fitness levels.

Teaching Tips

To succeed in fitness education, you must make many decisions—from selecting game formations to providing safe learning environments. Your awareness of these factors and the attention you give to each of them will determine your teaching success.

Management

Management refers to your ability to plan, organize, and direct. You need management skills in order to provide thoughtful, meaningful lessons. Your skills in planning lessons, moving students in and out of game formations, cueing students to start and stop, providing clear instructions, and arranging equipment are essential!

Planning: You must plan your lesson ahead of time. Consider your fitness goals and select activities to meet them. Consider the ages and skill levels of your students when planning the lesson.

Organization: Fitness games and activities should be designed to be continuous, so organize your lessons to provide smooth transitions between activities. To move from one game to the next without interrupting the flow of the lesson, you will need to plan the most effective and efficient ways to get the group into and out of formations. For example, if your students are in their personal space warming up with jump ropes, you must decide ahead of time how the ropes will be put away and how students will move into the next activity. You may have your students jog a lap and place their ropes over your extended arm as they pass by. Or you may choose four students to extend their arms so the others can return their jump ropes. As the students continue jogging, you can divide them into teams ready to play. (Quick ways to divide them into teams are by hair color, clothing color, or birthdays.)

Cues and Signals: You must be able to gain the attention of your students quickly when starting an activity or switching from one activity to another. Otherwise, their heart rates will drop and the children will no longer be working aerobically.

All teachers develop their own techniques for cueing their students to stop and listen for instructions. Call out a word such as "freeze," use a drum, or clap your hands. Whatever you decide on, establish it early, use it consistently, and reinforce it throughout the year. Taking time at the beginning of the year to teach your students cues will pay off later!

Giving Instructions: Always give students clear instructions so they know what they should be doing. Avoid lengthy directions or explanations, and use cue words so you are as clear and concise as possible. Cue words help students focus on the skill being taught. Consider what key information must be discussed in order for your students to play the game you have selected. Practice verbalizing the directions to yourself and see if they make sense to you. This will help you refine the instructions before you give them to your students.

Age Appropriateness

Consider the age level of your students. Do not try to introduce a new concept all at once. Build a strong understanding by teaching one concept at a time. For example, teaching children about target heart rates: First they must be able to locate their pulses. Next, the children need to understand that exercise makes the pulse go fast and rest slows the pulse down. After they understand this, they are ready to learn to count their pulses at rest and during exercise. Then introduce target heart rate. Explain how exercising within an appropriate heart rate range will make their hearts stronger and more efficient. Last, teach them how to calculate their target heart rates and monitor themselves during exercise.

Consider the skill level of your students. Do not expect children to play a game that includes skills you have not taught them. Do not require students to perform exercise tasks that are inappropriate for their age. It is unrealistic to expect first grade students to run a mile nonstop or to climb to the top of an 8-foot rope! Think about the activity you have selected. Trust your judgment. This decision-making process will become easier as you spend more and more time with your students.

Equipment

Our fitness games and activities may use several different pieces of equipment. Plan the physical placement and distribution of this equipment to save time and still provide a safe playing environment.

There are many simple yet effective ways to distribute equipment. One is to put students in squads, then call the squads one by one to get their equipment. Or the first person in each squad could get equipment for all of the squad members. Another way to distribute equipment is to pick a color and let students with that color in their shirts get their equipment. Continue selecting colors until all have whatever they need. Or call out a letter of the alphabet. Those students whose names begin with that letter may get their equipment. Keep calling out letters until everyone has been called. Other ways to distribute equipment are by birthday months, the number of brothers and sisters students have, and eye color.

Put equipment where it is easily accessible but out of the way until it is needed. Spread out equipment along the edge of the play area. For example, if you are using ribbons, balls, *and* beanbags, select a specific area for each type of equipment. Put each ribbon in its own space along the length of the wall, boxes of balls at another wall, and piles of beanbags at a third wall. This allows the participants to retrieve or deposit equipment without congestion.

We describe our games as though they are being played in gymnasiums, but a gym is not a necessity. Many of the games and activities may also be played out-of-doors. Make safety a primary concern when deciding if your play area is appropriate for a particular activity.

Safety

Teach students how to move safely in gyms and play areas. You cannot expect them to do this without proper instruction. Have young or inexperienced students practice moving in open spaces. Ask them to practice first at slow speeds. As their skills improve add other elements to the activity, such as changing speeds, changing directions, and using a variety of pathways (straight lines, zigzags, curves). Make this a game and have fun with it! Your students will become safe movers while they learn to be skilled movers.

Always consider the individual health concerns of your students. You can review school records or consult your school nurse to see if you have any students with special health problems. Work with the parents and child whenever you receive a note from home regarding a health concern. Select appropriate alternate activities, and invite the student to be part of the decision-making process.

For students with disabilities, you may modify the fitness activity or provide alternatives. By providing different equipment (lighter or larger balls, longer or shorter handles) and by adjusting your expectations, you can effectively adapt our games to meet individual needs. Fitness activities and programs that are self-paced also help integrate children with special needs into the physical education environment. Many of the games in this book allow self-pacing. Finally, you must consult parents and support people in order to provide safe learning activities for your students with disabilities. Special educators and assistants can offer many helpful suggestions for modifying a fitness program. The information they provide can help make your program a fun and rewarding learning experience for all students!

How to Use This Book

Fitness Fun is divided into three sections: warm-up, quick, and main activities. Each section contains learning activities that develop cardiorespiratory fitness, flexibility, muscular strength, and muscular endurance in children. Warm-ups are short duration activities used at the beginning of a lesson to prepare for more strenuous movement. Quick activities are designed to be used for short periods. These two kinds of activities should, together, last no longer than 10 minutes. The majority of a lesson should be made up of main activities chosen to meet the day's specific fitness objective.

Understanding the Fitness Symbols

Symbols representing each of the four fitness components show which fitness benefits each activity offers.

 represents cardiorespiratory fitness;

 represents muscular strength;

 represents muscular endurance; and

 represents flexibility.

The symbol for the principal fitness component that is enhanced by a game appears larger than the others.

Recommended grade ranges appear in the horizontal bar at the top of each game. Game formations and required equipment for each game are included on the game page. We also include hints and safety tips for some of the games. These may further assist you when you present activities to your students. Variations of some games are suggested to extend an activity.

11

Using the Game Finder

The game finder that follows is designed to help you locate games and activities quickly and easily. The fitness activities appear vertically and are listed alphabetically. The categories that appear horizontally will help you find games that meet your teaching needs; they include grade level, fitness components, and sport skills utilized in the activities. Remember, grade levels are *suggested* ranges. A capital letter (C, S, E, or F) indicates the principal fitness component developed in the activity. A lowercase c, s, e, or f indicates any secondary fitness component. The sport skills practiced in an activity are indicated by an abbreviation of the sport name. For an example of how to use the game finder, refer to the game Fitness Follow-the-Leader. This *quick activity* is recommended for play by students in *kindergarten through 5th grade*. It will improve *cardiorespiratory fitness* and help develop *muscular strength*. *No* particular *sport skills* are used.

Use the game finder to help you reach your teaching goals. Decide what areas of fitness you want to improve in your students and then select the activities that will best help you do this.

The material in *Fitness Fun* will help you achieve fitness success with children. Combine a positive attitude with your energy, enthusiasm, and belief that what you are doing is important, and you will motivate children to learn about fitness and commit themselves to living an active life. They will discover the joy in being active and will learn that exercise is fun and a rewarding experience that no one should go without!

Game Finder

Activity type

W = Warm-up
Q = Quick
M = Main

Primary fitness benefit

C = cardiorespiratory
S = muscular strength
E = muscular endurance
F = flexibility

Secondary fitness benefit

c = cardiorespiratory
s = muscular strength
e = muscular endurance
f = flexibility

Sport

B = baseball
Bb = basketball
Fb = football
F = frisbee
G = gymnastics
H = hockey
J = jump rope
R = racket sports
S = soccer
T = track
V = volleyball

(continued)

Game Finder *(continued)*

Game	Game number	Activity type	Page number	Grade range	Fitness benefits	Sport skills
All-Star Action	82	M	98	4-8	C,s	Bb,B
Alphabet Tag	24	Q	43	K-3	C	
Animal Action	65	M	76	K-3	S,e	
BEAR Tag	43	Q	56	2-4	C,s,e	
Bandage Tag	35	Q	49	1-4	C	
Beanbag Slide	56	Q	64	3-6	C,s,e	
Beast Hunter	34	Q	49	K-6	S,c	B
Boxer Short Tag	44	Q	56	2-5	C	
Breakaway Fitness	13	W	31	4-8	C,e	
Broomstick Stretch	42	Q	54	1-8	F,e	
Chalk Talk	12	W	30	4-8	C,s	T
Circle Leader Exercise	58	Q	65	3-8	S,e,c	
Circle Tag	55	Q	64	3-8	C	
Crab Soccer	72	M	84	1-5	S	S
Crazy Eight	5	W	23	2-6	S,e,c	
Cross-Country Run	15	W	33	4-8	C,e,s	T
Dog Pound	64	M	75	K-3	C	J
Double-Double	74	M	86	2-6	E,c	
Drum Stretches	4	W	22	K-6	F,c	G,T
ET, Phone Home	40	Q	53	1-4	C	
Everybody's It!	32	Q	48	K-6	C,s	
Figure Eight Fitness	17	W	35	4-8	C,s,e	T
Fit Stop	75	M	88	2-8	C,s,e,f	R,S, Bb,V, B,T, H,Fb, F,J
Fitness Circuit	60	Q	68	3-8	S,e,c	

	Game number	Activity type	Page number	Grade range	Fitness benefits	Sport skills
Fitness Course	68	M	80	K-8	C,s,e	G
Fitness Follow-the-Leader	29	Q	46	K-5	C,s	
Fitness Freedom	83	M	99	4-8	C,s	S,Bb,B,H
Flashcard Flexibility	16	W	34	5-8	F	
Flex-Stretch	19	W	37	5-8	F	G
Footloose	36	Q	50	K-8	C,s,e	
Four Corners	6	W	24	3-6	C,e	
Foxes and Hounds	57	Q	65	3-8	C	S,Bb,H
Fun Partner Relays	46	Q	58	2-6	C,s,e	
Garbage Aerobics	49	Q	60	3-5	S,c,f	
Getting-to-Know-You Jog	11	W	29	4-6	C,s,e	
Ghostbusters	27	Q	44	K-5	C	
Ghosting Around!	22	Q	42	K-2	C,s,e	
Go for Dough	66	M	78	K-5	C,s,e	
Great Jelly Bean Run	20	W	38	4-8	C,e	T
Guard Your Pin	77	M	90	3-8	S,c	H,S,B,F
Health Hopping	67	M	79	K-5	E,s	
Healthy Heart	41	Q	53	1-6	C	
Hideout	73	M	85	2-5	C,s	B,T
High Five Tag	48	Q	59	3-6	C	
Hoop Out	78	M	92	4-6	C	B,S
I Need to Stretch	8	W	26	3-6	F	
Icicle Tag	33	Q	48	K-6	C	
Jumping Jack Tag	50	Q	61	3-6	C,s,e	

(continued)

Game	Game number	Activity type	Page number	Grade range	Fitness benefits	Sport skills
Jumping Jacks, Jumping Jills, Angels in the Snow	3	W	21	K-3	E	
Jump Rope Stretch	10	W	28	3-8	F	J,G
"Ketchup" Tag	52	Q	62	3-6	C,s,e	T
Lily Pad Pond	25	Q	43	K-3	S,e	
Lott'ist Tod	7	W	25	3-6	C,e	
Mad Bomber	39	Q	52	1-5	C,s	S,H, Bb
Magic Carpets	28	Q	45	K-3	S	
Monkeys and Baboons	45	Q	57	2-6	C	
Mountain Trip	63	M	74	K-2	C	
Movement Fun	71	M	83	1-4	C,s,e,f	
Muscle Simon Says	61	Q	69	4-8	S,e	
Mystery Mover Champ	26	Q	44	1-3	C	
Partner Challenge	54	Q	63	3-8	C,s,e	
Patty Cake Polka	47	Q	59	2-6	C	
Pick-a-Task	2	W	20	K-6	F,s,c	
Picture a Pathway	30	Q	46	K-5	S,e	
Poison Poison	51	Q	61	3-6	C	B
Repeat Relays	69	M	81	K-6	C	
Rhymin' Rappin' and Stretchin'	9	W	27	3-6	F,c	
Rip City	62	Q	70	4-8	C	S,Bb
Scooter-Chute	79	M	93	4-6	S,e	
Sharks and Surfers	70	M	82	1-5	S,e	
Shower Ball	37	Q	51	K-6	C,e	B
Skating Rink Fitness	1	W	20	K-3	C,e	

Game number	Activity type	Page number	Grade range	Fitness benefits	Sport skills
Skipper's Delight	80	M	96	4-8	C,e	J
Snake Catcher	38	Q	52	1-4	C	
Star Trooper	53	Q	62	3-8	C	
Stop and Go	31	Q	47	K-5	E,s	
Strength Challenge	85	M	101	4-8	S,e	
Stretch Here, Stretch There	14	W	32	4-8	F,c	
Stretch Yourself	18	W	36	5-8	F	
Stretching Routine	21	W	39	4-8	F	G,T
Teddy Bear Stretch	23	Q	42	K-2	F	
They Work Hard for Their Sweat	59	Q	66	3-8	S,e,c	
Wacky-Ball	81	M	97	4-8	C	S
Water-Skiing	84	M	100	4-8	S,e	T
We Stretch, They Stretch	76	M	89	K-3	F,c	G

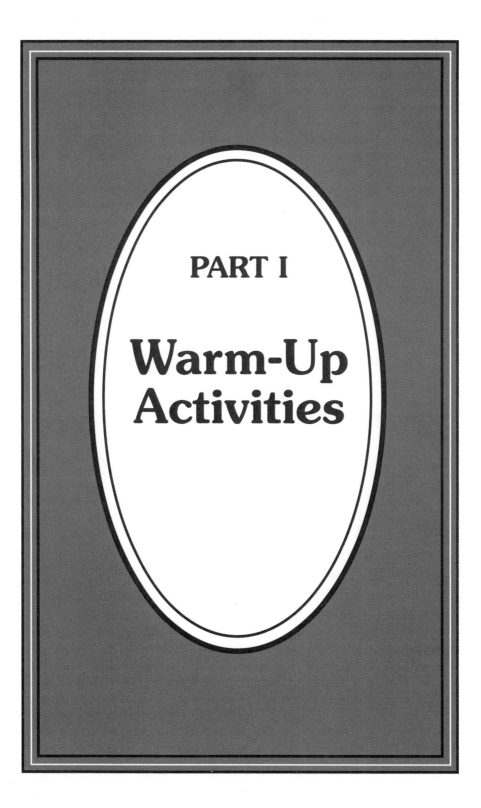

PART I

Warm-Up Activities

1. Skating Rink Fitness

K	1	2	3				

Equipment: Music

Formation: Personal space—this refers to the space around a child that allows room to move in place without contacting anyone or anything.

As students pretend they are skating, call out movements for them to perform throughout the gym. Try movements like these: Skate fast, skate slow; with a partner; backwards; in fours. Girls skate on the inside, boys on the outside; boys skate clockwise, girls counterclockwise. Skate a figure 8. Start and stop. Skate the letter *A*; the answer to 2 + 2; your name.

2. Pick-a-Task

K	1	2	3	4	5	6	

Equipment: 1 box of flexibility task cards (pelican stretch, straddle stretch, butterfly stretch), 1 box of locomotor task cards (crabwalk, bearwalk, seal-walk, and basic dance steps such as grapevine, polka, schottische); music

Formation: Personal space; boxes are in middle of gym

Have a student draw a card from the locomotor box and read it aloud. Students perform the task as the music plays; when the music stops the students freeze. The first student to freeze picks and reads a card from the flexibility box and the class does the exercise together. Continue until the students are warmed up.

3. Jumping Jacks, Jumping Jills, Angels in the Snow

K	1	2	3			Warm-up Activity

Equipment: Music

Formation: Personal space

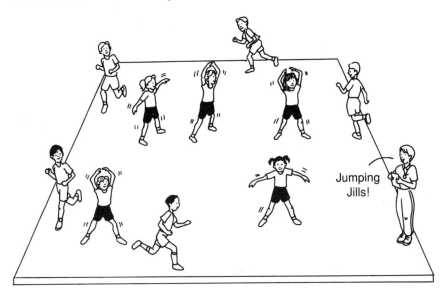

Jumping Jills!

Call out ways for students to move around the gym (skip, hop, gallop, jog, etc.). After a short period of movement, introduce jumping jacks and jumping jills: When you call jumping jacks, the boys do that exercise while the girls continue to travel; reverse the pattern when you call jumping jills. Then ask the class if anyone can do an angel in the snow: The students lie down and practice moving just their arms, then just their legs. Then combine arm and leg movements in various ways. After students understand each cue, have them move about the gym to your calls of jumping jacks, jumping jills, or angels in the snow.

4. Drum Stretches

K	1	2	3	4	5	6	

Warm-up Activity

Equipment: Drum

Formation: Personal space

Have students perform a variety of locomotor movements. Start the drum beat and call out a stretching exercise. Students hold the stretch for eight slow beats of the drum. They begin moving when the drum stops. Repeat the pattern several times using exercises such as long sit stretch, straddle stretch, figure four stretch, pelican stretch, butterfly stretch, calf stretch, bent elbow stretch, and cross chest stretch.

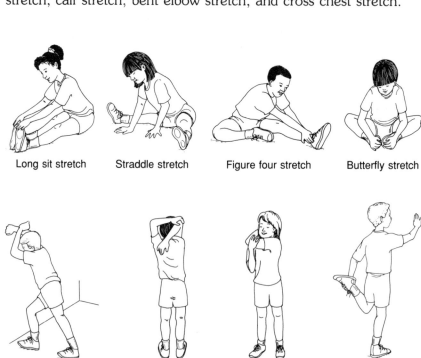

Long sit stretch Straddle stretch Figure four stretch Butterfly stretch

Calf stretch Bent elbow stretch Cross chest stretch Pelican stretch

5. Crazy Eight

Warm-
up
Activity

Equipment: Music or drum

Formation: Personal space

This is an exercise routine that takes eight counts. Play music that has a steady beat, or use a drum to count the beats. Students do steps 1 through 6, then repeat the pattern.

1. Use an alternating heel-toe pivot to move feet apart eight counts out and together eight counts in ("Out, 2, 3, 4, 5, 6, 7, 8; in, 2, 3, 4, 5, 6, 7, 8").
2. Touch head, shoulder, chest, waist, thighs, knees, toes, floor.
3. Walk alternating hands out on floor for eight counts into a push-up position.
4. Do eight push-ups.
5. Walk hands back in eight counts.
6. Straighten up and slap hands eight counts (like wiping hands off).
7. Repeat.

Variation: Use anatomical names for the muscles in step 2: deltoids ("delts") for shoulders, pectorals ("pecs") for chest, and quadriceps ("quads") for thighs.

6. Four Corners

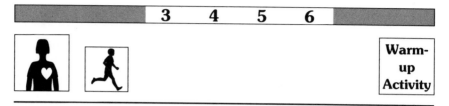
Equipment: 4 movement task signs, one in each corner of the gym; music

Formation: Students in 4 groups, one at each corner

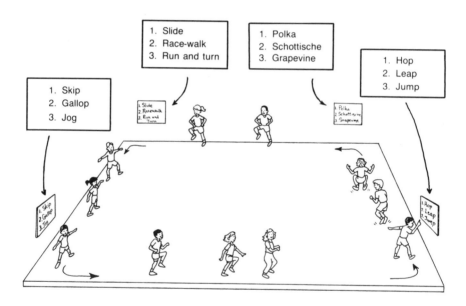

The students perform the first movement on their signs while traveling to the next corner, where they begin the first movement on that sign, and so on, as they progress from corner to corner. When they return to their starting corner, they begin the second movement listed and continue working their way through the lists around the gym until they have completed all of the tasks. Play music throughout the activity to motivate the class.

7. Lott' ist Tod

	3	4	5	6	

Equipment: Music, *"Lott' ist Tod"* record (RCA #45-6170)

Formation: Personal space along outside line of gym, facing center

This routine is adapted from the basic German dance *"Lott' ist Tod."*
Use the following cues to lead the activity.

1. Slide four slow steps left.
2. Slide eight fast steps right.
3. Repeat the two movements.
4. Turn left and run 16 steps.
5. Turn right and run 16 steps.
6. Repeat from the beginning until the song is over.

Hint: Help students by counting aloud, and have them count to
themselves so they will be ready to change directions. Practice re-
versing directions.

8. I Need to Stretch

3	4	5	6	

Equipment: 3-5 foam balls for 30 students; 4 cones

Formation: Personal space around the playing field; stretching area marked off by cones

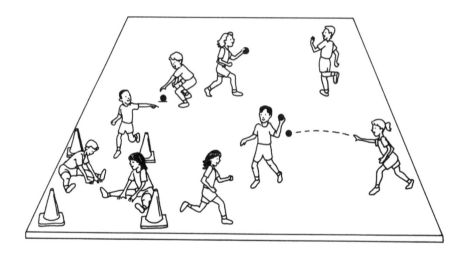

The foam balls are "tight muscle" balls and can be thrown by any student. Students who are hit must go to the stretching area and stretch for 30 seconds before reentering the game. Continue until the class is warmed up.

Hint: Some students may not get hit, so periodically signal the class to stop and perform specific stretches. Students learning stretches need visual aids. Post a chart with the pictures and names of the stretches (see page 22 for illustrations of the stretches). This will free you to manage the game.

9. Rhymin' Rappin' and Stretchin'

	3	4	5	6	

Equipment: Page of tongue twisters, rhymes, and raps for each student; music

Formation: Personal space

Each student holds a copy of the phrases while jogging. Stop the music and call out a stretching exercise (see page 22). While stretching, the students recite the first rhyme twice. Continue until students are warmed up. Here are some sample rhymes:

You can't sit and stay fit, so get in the groove and move!

Warmin' up can be fun, gotta flex before you run. So get down on the ground and stretch. Get down on the ground and stretch.

If you want to get in shape—JUST DO IT! If you want to stay in shape—STICK TO IT! Just do it! Stick to it! Just do it!

Hustle, hustle—work that muscle! Run, run—it's lots of fun!

Hint: If the students already know several stretches, play a musical tape with pauses dubbed in. Allow students to select their own stretches and raps each time the music stops.

10. Jump Rope Stretch

	3	4	5	6	7	8

Equipment: 1 jump rope for each student

Formation: Personal space

This activity incorporates a number of stretches using a jump rope. The students fold their ropes in half and hold them over their heads while standing with their feet in a straddle position. Use the following cues to lead the activity.

1. Bend right 2 times for 4 counts (keep the hips square). Use the following cues to lead the activity.
   Bend left 2 times for 4 counts.

2. Twist right 2 times for 4 counts.
   Twist left 2 times for 4 counts.

3. Slowly lower rope behind back, then bring it over head and lower it in front; keep arms straight. Do this 4 times.

4. Touch floor, keeping knees slightly bent. Do not bounce. Hold for 4 counts. Do this 4 times.

   The students sit on the floor in straddle position.

5. Stretch over the left leg 4 times for 4 counts. Stretch over the right leg 4 times for 4 counts.

6. Stretch forward 4 times for 4 counts.

   The students lie on their backs with their ropes around the bottom of one foot.

7. Begin with leg bent; straighten it 4 times for 4 counts. Repeat with other leg.

8. Begin with leg straight and on the floor; bring leg up as close to the head as possible 2 times for 4 counts. Repeat with other leg.

11. Getting-to-Know-You Jog

4   5   6

Warm-up Activity

Equipment: Pencils and questionnaire for each student; music

Formation: Personal space on the gym floor

"Getting-to-Know-You Jog" is a fun way to obtain information about your students. Knowing family information, individual interests, strengths, and weaknesses will help you understand your students and plan your lessons.

The students jog slowly around the gym while the music plays. When it stops, they go to their questionnaires, which they left on the floor, and answer the first question. When they finish question 1, they begin doing an exercise (jumping jacks, sit-ups, or push-ups). (This shows you when everyone is ready for another jog.) Continue this routine until the questionnaires are complete. Fun variations include jumping continuously around the gym, jogging with hands on knees, galloping with hands on hips, jogging or skipping backwards while looking over one shoulder, doing a grapevine step (step right with right foot, step right with left foot crossing over behind, step right with right foot, step right with left foot crossing over in front, and repeat) around the gym, racewalking, or jumping and touching the basketball hoop.

12. Chalk Talk

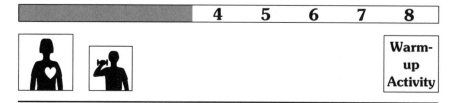

Warm-up Activity

Equipment: Chalkboard, chalk; music; 4 cones

Formation: 1 cone set on each corner of gym; chalkboard near but safely outside jogging lane; instructor by chalkboard; students around perimeter of gym

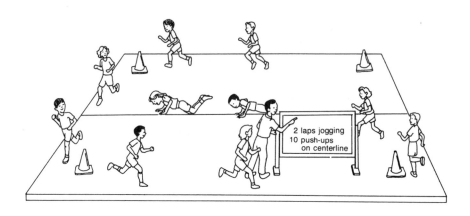

2 laps jogging
10 push-ups
on centerline

Students start jogging around the gym outside the cones. Each time they pass the chalkboard they read an exercise task they are to do. Add a new exercise each time the students complete a lap. If you do not wish to add anything new, have the students continue doing the last task. Or give the chalk to different students and let them write down their favorites!

Exercise tasks might include jogging 2 laps; galloping 1 lap; doing 10 push-ups on the centerline; jogging the sidelines; seal-walking the endlines; racewalking 1 lap; doing 15 stomach crunches on the centerline; or "Your choice!"

13. Breakaway Fitness

		4	5	6	7	8	

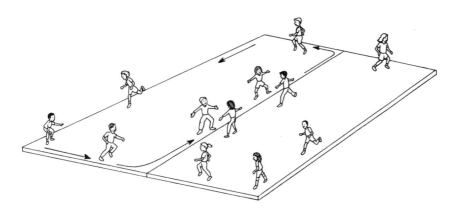

Warm-
up
Activity

Equipment: Music

Formation: Students in pairs, lined up single file across the gym from one another

The first pair of partners jog toward the centerline, face each other, and begin the same locomotor movement or pattern down the center lane of the gym. The entire class follows down the center lane copying the leaders' movement. When they reach the endline, partners break away and jog down their own sidelines. The leaders repeat their movement, which ends their "turn" and brings the next pair into position. The new leaders then perform a different movement for the class to follow.

Movements could include basketball slides (knees bent, hands in defensive position, move sideways), grapevine steps, jogging backwards, skipping and clapping, "jump, jump, clap, clap" (jump forward two jumps, clap in place twice; repeat to endline), and jogging while tapping the head with one hand and rubbing the stomach with the other.

Hint: Remember to keep students moving throughout the entire activity so they maintain their target heart rates.

14. Stretch Here, Stretch There

	4	5	6	7	8

Warm-
up
Activity

Equipment: Signs with stretching exercises written on them (see page 22)

Formation: Signs taped on the walls around gym; students evenly positioned at the signs

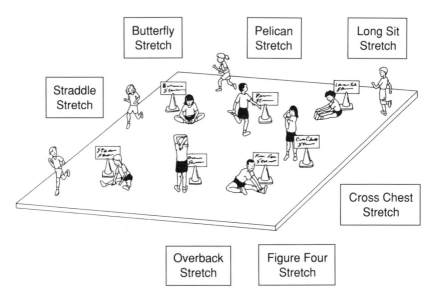

Students perform the stretching exercise at their station for 1 to 2 minutes. Then they jog 2 laps around the gym. When they complete their laps, they jog to the next station, do the stretching exercise, and jog 2 laps. The students continue stretching and jogging until they complete the circuit.

Safety Tip:

If you need to provide room for safe jogging, tape the stretching signs to cones and move them to the middle of the play area.

15. Cross-Country Run

		4	5	6	7	8

Warm-up Activity

Equipment: Instruction sheet; 1 beanbag or yarn ball for each student

Formation: Students gathered near instructor

Give student a sheet of instructions with a description of a cross-country run on it, for example:

1. Jog across the soccer field.
2. Jog to the furthest goal.
3. Jump and touch the goalpost three times.
4. Jog to the basketball hoop.
5. Jog to the baseball field and run the bases.
6. Jog to the box under the tree.
7. Take a beanbag or yarn ball from the box and return it to your teacher.

Students go off individually and do the run in the specified area.

Hint: This is a *sample* cross-country run. When you write your own, use the facilities and outdoor equipment available to you. Incorporate any equipment, such as slides, monkey bars, and balance beams, that may be on your playground. Younger students will need more time to run the course.

16. Flashcard Flexibility

	5	6	7	8

Equipment: 1 set of stretching cards per group (stretching cards have names of muscles on one side and functions on the other)

Formation: Groups of 5-6 students

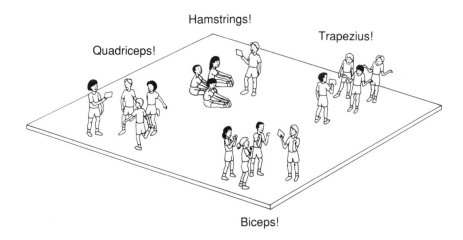

Quadriceps! Hamstrings! Trapezius! Biceps!

Choose one student in each group to be a leader and give each a set of stretching cards. Each group leader draws a card and calls out a muscle's function. The group members identify the muscle and do the appropriate stretch. For example, the leader draws the card *quadriceps*. The leader reads, "the muscle that straightens the leg." Participants respond, "Quadriceps," and all then stretch their quadriceps. The leader continues selecting cards until all the major muscles are stretched.

Examples of other muscle functions are hamstrings, bend the leg; biceps, bend the arm; triceps, straighten the arm; gastrocnemius (calf), extend the ankle; gluteals, extend the hip; deltoids, move the arm up, forward, and back; trapezius, raise the shoulders.

17. Figure Eight Fitness

			4	**5**	**6**	**7**	**8**

			Warm-up Activity

Equipment: 8 cones; music

Formation: Cones in large figure eight

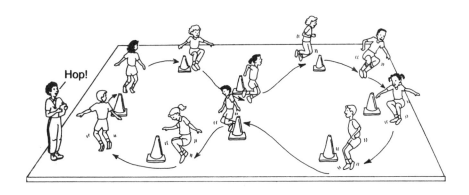

Students move single file around the cones while performing the locomotor movements that you call out, such as skip, hop, gallop, crabwalk, bearwalk, grapevine, polka, and racewalk. Encourage students to keep moving throughout the entire activity to maintain their target heart rates.

18. Stretch Yourself

		5	6	7	8

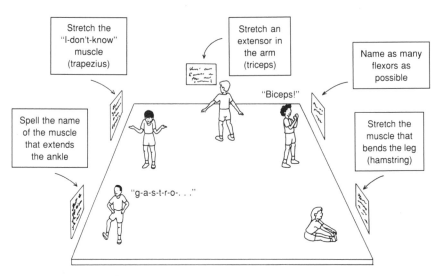

Warm-up Activity

Equipment: Signs with a stretching task (see p. 22) written on each one

Formation: Signs posted on the walls; students evenly dispersed among the different stations

Stretch the "I-don't-know" muscle (trapezius)

Stretch an extensor in the arm (triceps)

Name as many flexors as possible

"Biceps!"

Spell the name of the muscle that extends the ankle

Stretch the muscle that bends the leg (hamstring)

"g-a-s-t-r-o-. . ."

Students move from station to station completing the stretching exercises. They may move freely, or you may signal them to rotate to the next station at 1-minute intervals.

Stretching tasks include stretching the muscle that bends the leg (hamstring); stretching an extensor in the arm (triceps); spelling the name of the muscle that extends the ankle (gastrocnemius) then stretching it; stretching the "I-don't-know" muscle (trapezius); stretching the gluteals; naming as many flexors as possible (biceps, hamstring); and stretching the gastrocnemius two different ways.

Hint: This activity is best done *after* students have learned the names of the muscles and proper stretching exercises for each of them.

19. Flex-Stretch

	5	6	7	8

Equipment: Surgical tubing, dowels, jump ropes, towels

Formation: Students in 4 groups; each type of equipment in a separate area of gym

This activity should not be done until students have learned the proper way to perform specific stretches.

Students use the equipment in stretching exercises at each station. Groups spend 2 minutes at each area and then rotate to the next. Encourage the students to stretch through the full range of motion, create new stretches, and stretch with a partner.

Using any one of the four kinds of equipment, students stand with their feet in a straddle position and extend their arms over their heads.

1. Bend right 2 times for 4 counts (keep the hips square).
   Bend left 2 times for 4 counts.
2. Twist right 2 times for 4 counts.
   Twist left 2 times for 4 counts.
3. Slowly lower hands behind back as far as possible, then bring them over head and lower them in front; do this 4 times (keep arms straight).
4. Keeping knees slightly bent, bend forward and touch floor. Do not bounce. Hold for 4 counts. Repeat 3 more times.

20. Great Jelly Bean Run

		4	5	6	7	8

Warm-up Activity

Equipment: 1 notecard, 1 Zip-lock bag, and 1 name label for each student; 4 cones; marking pen

Formation: 1 cone on each corner of playing area; students along the periphery of the gym

The Great Jelly Bean Run is a unique fitness activity. We are not advocating candy as a healthy snack; we are using it as a "novel" motivator. Each student's task is to jog as many laps as possible in a given period. The duration will depend on individual class periods. Students should jog two or three times each week.

Students carry their notecards, which have their names on them, as they begin jogging laps around the cones. As students pass you, put dots on their cards with a marking pen. When the jogging time has ended, collect the cards and count the dots. This can be done relatively quickly as the cards are handed in, or students may tally their own dots. Write the totals on their cards. After class, put the totals in a Jelly Bean Run record book containing class lists for all the classes participating in the run. At the end of the week, or daily, put the same number of jelly beans as laps run in each student's jelly bean bag. Give the students their bags of jelly beans when the Great Jelly Bean Run has ended. They may either eat the jelly beans or use them like tokens to trade for outside play or the use of equipment during recess.

Hint: Teachers who do not want to use jelly beans can use peanuts or macaroni pieces for tokens.

21. Stretching Routine

		4	5	6	7	8

Warm-up Activity

Equipment: Music (slow, for stretching)

Formation: Personal space

Everyone slowly stretches to the beat of the music.

The following are examples of basic stretching routines (see page 22 for stretching positions).

Long sit position: Flex and extend ankles (8 counts); circle right ankle (4 times clockwise, 4 times counterclockwise); circle left ankle (4 times clockwise, 4 times counterclockwise).

Seated straddle position: Stretch right (4 counts); stretch center (4 counts); stretch left (4 counts); repeat (4 times).

Seated butterfly position: Stretch spine up, gently push knees to the ground 4 times; then bend at waist and bring chest to feet 4 counts; repeat (4 times).

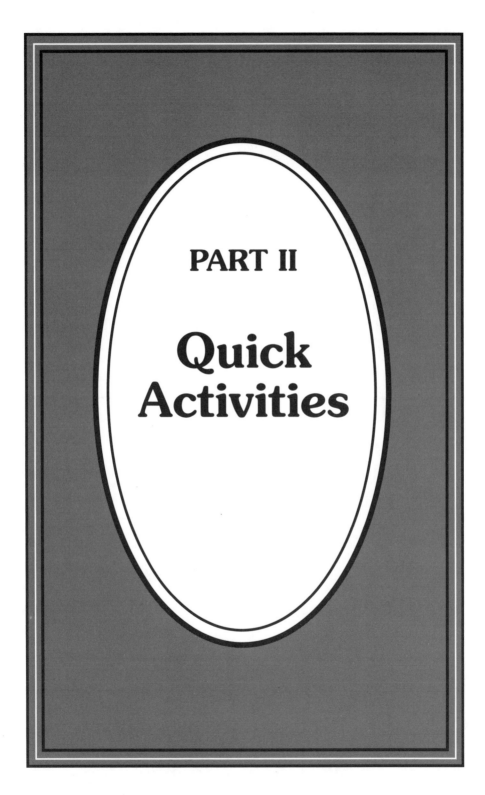

PART II

Quick
Activities

22. Ghosting Around!

K	1	2	

Equipment: 1 "Ghosting Around" bag (brown paper bag); "Ghostbuster" music; movement messages shaped like ghosts

Formation: Personal space

From your bag labeled "Ghosting Around," a student draws a ghost-shaped message and reads it aloud. (You may read cards for younger students.) The students move around the gym performing the movement while you play the song "Ghostbusters." When the music stops, students freeze and await the next movement message.

Ghostbuster messages might include these: Gallop around the gym; fly like a ghost; tiptoe quickly and quietly around the gym; do 10 "ghost sit-ups" (regular sit-ups).

23. Teddy Bear Stretch

K	1	2	

Equipment: Stuffed teddy bear

Formation: Personal space

Face your students while holding the teddy bear, and manipulate the bear's body parts into a variety of stretches. The students follow along and repeat what the bear is doing.

This is an excellent cool-down activity and a nice way to get students on the floor and ready for relaxation exercises before ending the class.

Refer to page 22 for stretching exercises.

24. Alphabet Tag

K	1	2	3	

Quick Activity

Equipment: None

Formation: Personal space

Choose four students to be "it." When an "it" tags someone, that person freezes into the shape of a letter. As soon as another player guesses the letter, the tagged person may go back into the game. Choose new taggers frequently.

Variation: The tagger tells the person tagged what letter to form.

25. Lily Pad Pond

K	1	2	3	

Quick Activity

Equipment: 1 hoop per student, 5 extra hoops

Formation: Hoops scattered on the floor represent lily pads, some close together and others far apart to present different jumping distances

Children pretend they are frogs and move about in the "pond" by jumping from lily pad to lily pad (the hoops). If players land in the water they must quickly get onto a pad by "swimming" to it. Players may imitate swimming in fast, moderate, or slow speeds. Encourage players to share lily pads with each other.

43

26. Mystery Mover Champ

1	**2**	**3**		

Quick Activity

Equipment: Music (Phyllis Weikart's "Rhythmically Moving #5" works well); 10-15 cards marked "Mystery Mover Champ"

Formation: Personal space

Have students close their eyes and listen to a piece of music. Ask them to think about how the music makes them feel and how they could move to the music. Let students move to the music. Choose 2 or 3 creative students and give each a Mystery Mover Champ card. (This helps motivate students to be creative.) Mystery mover champs demonstrate their movement ideas one at a time and all of the students try each movement.

27. Ghostbusters

K	**1**	**2**	**3**	**4**	**5**	

Quick Activity

Equipment: None

Formation: 1-3 students (taggers) in middle of gym; remaining students (runners) at one endline

The runners (ghosts) yell, "Who you gonna call?" The taggers (ghostbusters) answer, "Ghostbusters!" The ghosts then attempt to run to the opposite endline without being tagged. Ghostbusters may leave the centerline to tag ghosts as they pass by. Those tagged become ghostbusters and gather on the centerline for the next run. Continue until all ghosts are caught. The last ghost caught can be the first ghostbuster for the new game.

Variation: Use a Teenage Mutant Ninja Turtle theme. The Shredders call out "Dudes," and the turtles yell "Cowabunga!"

28. Magic Carpets

Equipment: 1 carpet square for each student

Formation: Personal space; carpet squares upside down on floor

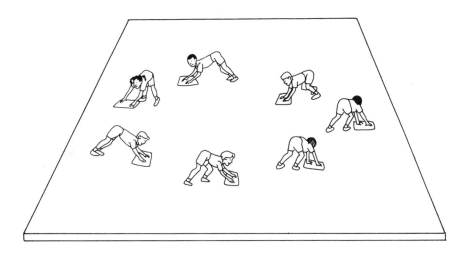

Tell students that the carpets are magic. Tell them all to lie stomach down on their carpets and then pull themselves forward; move backward; and turn around in a circle. Repeat these moves while sitting, then kneeling. It is also fun to do the "twist" while sitting, kneeling, and standing on the squares. Let students try to "drive" the carpets around the gym by placing their hands on the squares, lifting their hips in the air, and pushing on the floor with their feet. (Only older students should drive because younger children are not strong enough.)

Safety Tip:

Make sure students drive in the same direction.

45

29. Fitness Follow-the-Leader

K	1	2	3	4	5	

Quick Activity

Equipment: None

Formation: Students in single file

Choose one student to lead the line. As the leader travels around the gym using any type of movement (gallop, skip, grapevine step, crabwalk, jump, hop), the other students follow and copy the movement. The leader may add arm or leg movements while leading the line and may stop the group to do exercises such as push-ups, mountain climbers, and sit-ups. Select new leaders periodically, or select several leaders to lead smaller groups. This game is fun to play out-of-doors.

30. Picture a Pathway

K	1	2	3	4	5	

Quick Activity

Equipment: None

Formation: Students in pairs, one partner in front of the other, in two lines along one side of gym

Each person in the first line performs a task across the gym. When a student crosses the centerline, his or her partner begins the same task. Call out each activity, or place a list of tasks on the wall where students can read it and choose a task. Or let them make up their own. Examples include jump forward, jump to the side, jump forward, repeat; jump to the side 3 times, jump forward 2 times, repeat; jump forward 2 times, jump back, repeat; hop forward on right foot 4 times, hop forward on left foot 4 times, repeat.

31. Stop and Go

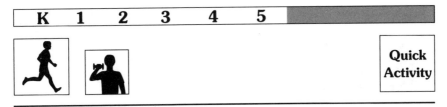

Quick Activity

Equipment: 10 STOP and 25 GO paper plates (GO plates each have a number from 1 to 10)

Formation: Personal space, each student standing by a paper plate

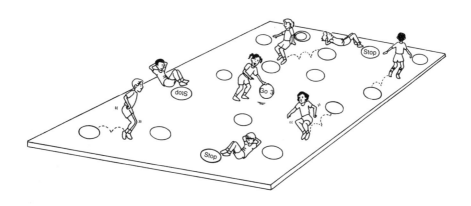

Place all plates face down on the gym floor. Choose a locomotor movement (skip, jump, gallop, leap, or hop) for children to use while traveling from plate to plate. Each student turns a plate over, reads it, performs the movement or exercise you have selected, and then replaces the plate face down. A "GO 3" plate means to jump (or skip, gallop, etc.) three times to another plate. If the student does not reach another plate within the number of jumps indicated, he or she may walk to a plate. A STOP plate means do 10 sit-ups (or push-ups, stretches, etc.) and then walk to another plate. This game can be played continuously, and you may change locomotor movements and exercises during the game.

32. Everybody's It!

K	1	2	3	4	5	6	

Quick
Activity

Equipment: None

Formation: Personal space

Everyone is "it." When students are tagged, they must move out of the play area and perform an exercise. If two people tag each other at the same time, they both move out. The game is over when there are only two students left. This game ends quickly so students should not have to wait long before it begins again.

33. Icicle Tag

K	1	2	3	4	5	6	

Quick
Activity

Equipment: 2 foam balls (freezers)

Formation: Personal space

Two students are chosen to be "it" and each is given a foam ball. (Younger students tag with the ball; older students may throw it.) When tagged, a student becomes an "icicle" and stands still, legs in a wide straddle position. A student can be unfrozen by a "sun," that is, any student who crawls through an icicle's legs. If a sun is tagged while crawling he or she becomes an icicle. Change "it"'s often.

34. Beast Hunter

K	1	2	3	4	5	6	

Quick Activity

Equipment: 12 yarn balls for every 25 students; 4 hockey sticks

Formation: Personal space

Four students are chosen to be beast hunters. Younger students ride their horses (hockey sticks); older students hunt on foot. All carry ammunition (yarn balls) to throw. The remaining students are "beasts." When beasts are hit, they lie down on their backs and raise their arms and legs straight up off the ground until all beasts have been hit. (Holding the "dead beast" position strengthens the stomach muscles.) The game starts again with new beast hunters.

35. Bandage Tag

	1	2	3	4	

Quick Activity

Equipment: None

Formation: Personal space

Everyone is "it." Each child may be tagged a total of three times but he or she must cover with one hand each area touched until the third tag. For example, if a student is first tagged on the elbow, she must hold or cover her elbow. If the second tag is on the back, she must also cover that area. Students are "frozen" on the third tag and move off the play area until the game begins again. The game moves quickly so you may want to play it several times.

36. Footloose

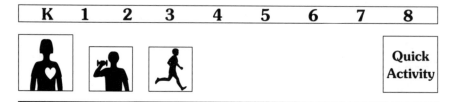

K	1	2	3	4	5	6	7	8

Quick
Activity

Equipment: Upbeat music (the song "Footloose" is appropriate); 1 towel for each student

Formation: Personal space, leader at front of room

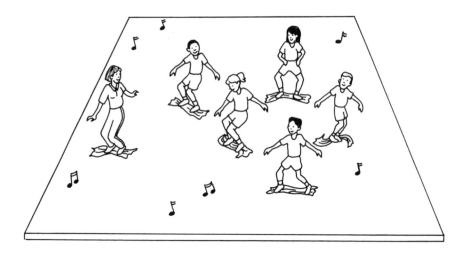

This activity introduces a new exercise tool, a towel. You may create movements to fit the music or design complete routines. Or let students invent their own moves.

Try these movements: Place the towel on the floor and stand with one foot on each end. Now twist (the towel lets your feet move with less friction); skate forward, then backward; do a forward scissors (shuffle feet forward and backward); do a straddle (move your feet apart, then together); twist to the right, to the left. Sitting on the towel, scoot forward, back, and sideways; spin with your knees tucked up and feet off the ground; spin turning right, turning left; alternately bend and extend your legs while moving your arms forward and back like a rowing machine.

37. Shower Ball

Quick Activity

Equipment: Small foam ball for each student

Formation: 2 teams positioned opposite each other along the centerline; balls scattered on the floor

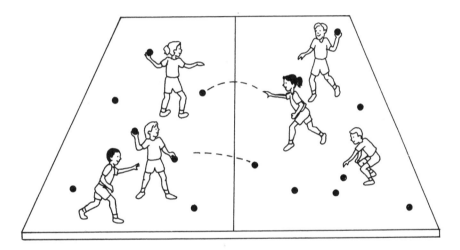

Each team tries to get rid of the foam balls on its side of the floor by throwing them to the other side. Call out "shower ball" to begin the game. Teams continue throwing until you call out "freeze." No balls may be thrown after the signal. Team members gather the balls on their side and count them. The team with the fewest balls wins. Give a second signal, and everyone starts throwing balls again.

Variation: This game can be played using hockey skills and sticks and pucks instead of balls, or as a soccer drill (no hands, kicking only).

Safety Tip:

Do not allow students to swing hockey sticks above their waists.

---

38. Snake Catcher

| 1 | 2 | 3 | 4 |

Quick Activity

Equipment: One jump rope for each group

Formation: Area divided into 4-6 squares; one group of 4-5 students in each square

Give one student (the snake) in each group a rope to drag on the floor. On your signal, the other players in the group try to catch the dragging end of the rope *in their hands*; do not allow players to step on the rope. When a player catches the rope, he or she becomes the snake. Remind snakes to watch where they are going. They must stay within their own areas.

39. Mad Bomber

| 1 | 2 | 3 | 4 | 5 |

Quick Activity

Equipment: 1 playground ball for each student

Formation: Personal space

Give each student a ball, then choose one to three students to be "Mad Bombers." The other students (dribblers) try to dribble close to their bodies to protect their balls from the bombers. Mad bombers attempt to throw and hit other players' balls with their own. Any dribbler whose ball is hit becomes a mad bomber until all of the balls have been hit.

Variations: When their balls are hit, players must go to the sideline and do an exercise before returning to the game.

Older students may play this game using hockey and soccer skills.

40. ET, Phone Home

1 2 3 4

Quick
Activity

Equipment: 3 "zappers" (foam pipes 1-2 feet long); ET music

Formation: Personal space

Choose three students to be "it" and give each a zapper. When the music begins, everyone starts moving. The taggers try to zap (touch, not hit) the other students (ETs) with their zappers. Zapped ETs freeze and hold their index fingers in the air. Other ETs may unfreeze zapped ones by touching their index fingers together as both students say, "ET, phone home."

41. Healthy Heart

1 2 3 4 5 6

Quick
Activity

Equipment: 3 foam balls labeled *TV*, *Fats*, and *Sugars*; 1 larger foam ball or throwing disk (to represent a healthy heart)

Formation: Personal space

This game dramatizes the effects of poor nutrition and a sedentary lifestyle on the heart. Explain to the students that too much sugar, fats, and TV are not good for the heart but that exercise *is* good and will make the heart stronger. Give a labeled ball to each of three students; they will throw to hit other players. Give the heart ball (or disk) to another student. If students get hit by one of the balls marked *Sugar*, *Fats*, or *TV*, they must freeze and call out "Healthy Heart, I need exercise!" The person with the healthy heart ball runs and tags the frozen players who are calling out and frees them to continue playing.

42. Broomstick Stretch

	1	2	3	4	5	6	7	8

Quick
Activity

Equipment: 1 3-foot dowel for each student; music

Formation: Personal space

Using the following instructions, guide students through these stretches *slowly*.

Overhead Stretch: "Stand with your feet shoulder-width apart, stretch and bring the dowel above your head. Relax your shoulders, keep your spine long and straight, and flex your knees. Now stretch forward from the hips. Your arms, spine, and pelvis should be parallel to the floor. Slowly roll up to the starting position."

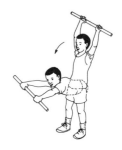

Forward Stretch: "Bend at the waist and hold the dowel behind your hips with the palms of your hands facing back. Move the dowel up and away from your hips toward your shoulders. Slowly straighten your spinal column and lower the dowel back to your hips."

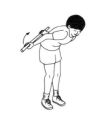

Torso Twists: "Place the dowel across your shoulders behind your neck. Hold it with your hands spread wide apart and your palms facing forward. Slowly twist your upper body to the right, then to the left."

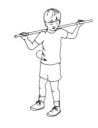

Side Dips: "Hold the dowel overhead with your arms stretched outward. Keep your legs slightly bent and let your upper body bend to the side from the hips." Do this toward both sides.

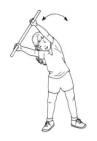

Step Overs: "Hold the dowel near each end in front of your body and step over it. Bring the dowel behind your back as far as you can without letting go. Now, lower the dowel, step over it again, and bring it back to its original position."

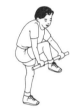

Achilles Stretch: Place the end of the dowel on the ground in front of you. Put one foot in front of the other while keeping your back foot straight. Bend your forward knee as much as you can while keeping your back heel on the ground."

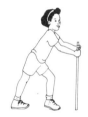

Side Leg Stretch: "Stand with your feet apart. Grasp one end of the dowel with both hands and place the other end on the ground at arms-length in front of one knee. Keep your other leg straight, and do a side lunge with a straight back."

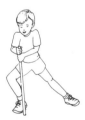

Hint: Make this activity fun! Use music and have the students follow you. Or choreograph a whole routine using all the stretches.

43. BEAR Tag
(Be Enthusiastic About Reading!)

2   3   4

Quick Activity

Equipment: Set of exercise task bear cards

Formation: Personal space

Four students are bears who try to tag the others. Tagged students get a bear card from the instructor and do the exercise written on it. Once completed, students return the bear cards and rejoin the game. Select new bears often.

Task cards might say do 5 push-ups, jump rope 1 minute, jump and reach 10 times, do 15 wall push-ups, do 10 sit-ups, or crabwalk across the gym.

Variation: For young students, bear hats made of construction paper and worn by the taggers add excitement. Use picture cards for younger students who cannot read.

44. Boxer Short Tag

2   3   4   5

Quick Activity

Equipment: 4-6 pairs of boxer shorts

Formation: Personal space

Choose four to six students to be "it." These students wear the boxer shorts. When they tag someone, that person becomes "it" and must put on the boxer shorts the tagger was wearing.

> **Safety Tip:**
> Have the students take off and put on the boxer shorts near the sideline.

45. Monkeys and Baboons

Quick Activity

Equipment: Scarves or flags for half the class

Formation: 2 groups: one with scarves, one without

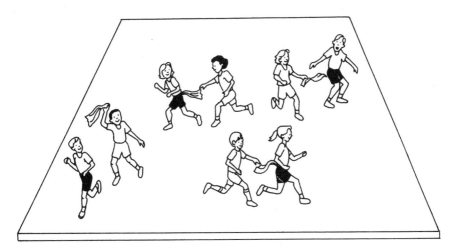

Explain that monkeys have tails (scarves tucked in at their waists) and baboons do not. The baboons get tails by pulling the scarves away from the monkeys. Monkeys who lose their tails become baboons, and the game continues.

46. Fun Partner Relays

Quick Activity

Equipment: None

Formation: Students paired, one behind the other, in double-line along one side of gym

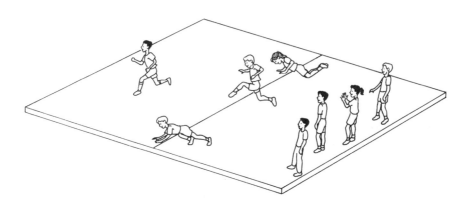

Those in the front line choose exercise movements and perform them across the gym and back. Those in the second line then copy their partners' movements. For example, a student might gallop to the centerline, do 5 mountain climbers (push-up position with one leg extended and one pulled up to chest, quickly alternate legs), and then gallop to the other side; skip to the centerline, roll once, then skip to other side; run to the centerline, leap once, and run to other side; or jog to the centerline, do 5 push-ups, then jog to other side. Have partners take turns making up and copying each other's exercise movements. Challenge older students to invent more difficult, complex activities.

47. Patty Cake Polka

	2	3	4	5	6	

Quick
Activity

Equipment: Recording of "Little Brown Jug"

Formation: Students in pairs facing each other, holding hands; pairs spaced throughout the gym

The students begin the dance mirroring each other. Cue the steps as follows:

1. Heel, toe, heel, toe, slide, slide, slide [point direction]
2. Heel, toe, heel, toe, slide, slide, slide [point in opposite direction]
3. Again! (repeat 1 & 2)
4. Reverse! (begin with opposite foot and repeat 1-3)
5. Clap right, clap left, clap both, clap knees
6. Right elbow swing & left elbow swing (or do a two-handed swing)

Repeat 1-6 throughout the song.

48. High Five Tag

	3	4	5	6	

Quick
Activity

Equipment: None

Formation: Personal space

Choose three students to be taggers. When students are tagged, they freeze with one hand high in the air. As soon as someone gives them a high five on their outstretched hands, they may rejoin the game. Select new taggers frequently.

49. Garbage Aerobics

3   4   5

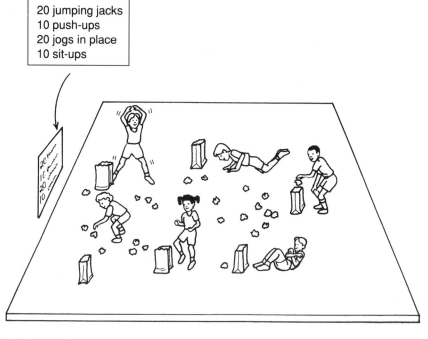

Quick Activity

Equipment: 1 grocery bag and 10 scrap paper balls for each student; music; exercise poster

Formation: Personal space with bags in front of students

> 20 jumping jacks
> 10 push-ups
> 20 jogs in place
> 10 sit-ups

Students do the exercise tasks listed on the poster and collect a paper ball for each completed task. They work their way through the list until all the "garbage" is gone then count the number of pieces each collected.

The exercise list might include 20 jumping jacks, 10 push-ups, 20 jogs in place, and 10 sit-ups. Repeat the exercises.

50. Jumping Jack Tag

	3	4	5	6	

Equipment: 3 pinnies for every 25 students

Formation: Personal space

Select two or three people to be "it" and give them pinnies to wear so that they can be distinguished from the other students. Because there are no safe bases, if students want to stop running ("rest") and not be tagged, they must do jumping jacks. Periodically change the exercise to be done while resting; for example, try sit-ups, wall push-ups, bleacher step-ups, and skier jumps. Tagged students trade places with the chasers who tagged them.

51. Poison Poison

	3	4	5	6	

Equipment: 3 foam balls, 2 the same color

Formation: Personal space

Roll the balls onto the floor. The same-colored balls are the poison balls and the other is the magic ball. Students pick up the poison balls and throw them at each other trying to hit below the waist. Players hit by poison balls must sit down and wait for someone to throw them the magic ball. They must catch the magic ball, stand up, and then throw the ball to another student who has been hit and is sitting down. If a poison ball hits the person holding the magic ball, that person must sit down and throw the ball to someone else.

52. "Ketchup" Tag

	3	4	5	6	

Equipment: None

Formation: Students in a large circle

Have students count off by fours, then call a number from one through four. Students assigned that number step outside the circle and run counterclockwise, trying to tag the person in front of them before they get back to their places. Remind students that they are being chased and to tag gently. Tagged students go to the center of the circle and do an exercise task that you give them; for example, 15 jumping jacks, 5 push-ups, 5 mountain climbers, or 5 sit-ups. The students may rejoin the circle when they have completed the task. Continue calling out numbers while the tagged students are performing their tasks.

53. Star Trooper

	3	4	5	6	7	8	

Quick Activity

Equipment: 4 foam balls

Formation: Personal space

Select four children to be star troopers; the others are aliens. The star troopers throw the balls at the aliens. When aliens are hit they are frozen until another player rescues them by giving them a high five. Continue playing for 1 to 2 minutes then have the star troopers select other students to replace them. Continue the game until all have been star troopers.

54. Partner Challenge

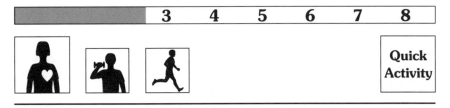

	3	4	5	6	7	8

Quick Activity

Equipment: None

Formation: Students in pairs lined up facing each other on opposite sides of gym

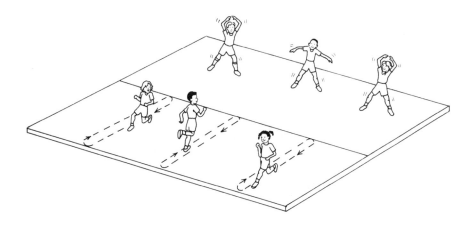

A partners run to the centerline and back to their spots for 30 seconds nonstop while B partners do jumping jacks on the sideline. Students count the number of times they do their tasks. After 30 seconds, partners meet on the centerline and tell each other their totals. When they go back to their own spots, they do what their partners had done. For example, A partners now do jumping jacks, and B partners run back and forth from the centerline to the sideline.

Ideas for partner tasks include sit-ups and jumping rope, crabwalk and stomach crunches, bearwalk and sit-ups, and mountain climbers and stomach crunches.

55. Circle Tag

	3	4	5	6	7	8

Quick Activity

Equipment: None

Formation: Students in groups of 4: 3 in a circle holding hands, 1 standing outside the circle

The person outside the circle is "it" and announces whom he or she will tag. The students forming the circle try to prevent the person from being caught by rotating their circle clockwise or counterclockwise. When a tag is made, the tagger and the taggee exchange places. The new tagger always tries to touch a person who has not been chased. The tagger may not reach over or under the circle to make a tag.

56. Beanbag Slide

	3	4	5	6	

Quick Activity

Equipment: 1 beanbag or small foam ball for each student

Formation: 2 teams, one on each side of play area

Place an equal number of beanbags on the floor on each side of the play area. On your signal, players slide beanbags (using their hands) toward the opposing team and attempt to hit each other's feet. Players hit by beanbags go to their sidelines and do 5 push-ups or 5 sit-ups. Then they may rejoin the game.

57. Foxes and Hounds

	3	4	5	6	7	8

Quick Activity

Equipment: Soccer balls for half the class

Formation: Students paired according to ability

One student in each pair is a fox and the other is a hound. The foxes have soccer balls that they dribble. The hounds attempt to retrieve the ball using basic soccer skills. A hound who successfully retrieves a ball becomes the fox and the other person becomes the hound.

This game may be played either one student versus another or a group of hounds against a group of foxes.

58. Circle Leader Exercise

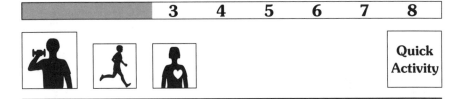

	3	4	5	6	7	8

Quick Activity

Equipment: Music; strength exercise poster

Formation: Students in 3 large circles

One student stands at the center of each circle and calls out strength exercises for that group to perform, referring to the list of strength exercises (push-ups, jumping jacks, sit-ups) if needed. The student leaders have the responsibility to keep everyone moving!

Variation: Leaders may do aerobic dance movements instead of strength exercises. After each movement, a new leader moves into the middle and leads an exercise keeping time to the music. Allow students to pass if they do not want to lead.

59. They Work Hard for Their Sweat

| | | | 3 | 4 | 5 | 6 | 7 | 8 |

Quick Activity

Equipment: Upbeat music (Donna Summer's "She Works Hard for the Money," Mercury record 812370-7); 2 benches

Formation: Students in 4 equal groups, together, they should form a square shape. (Have each group stand on one of the following markings: centerline, sideline, endline, sideline.)

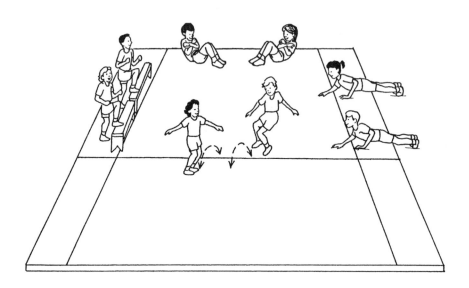

When the music begins, each group performs an exercise designed just for that line.

Line 1: Step-ups: The students step up on the bench with one foot, up with the other foot, down with the first foot, down with the second foot. Cue them with "up, up, down, down." If you do not have steps or benches, have the students do mountain climbers.

Line 2: Side jumps (skiers): The students stand next to the line and jump from side to side over the line.

Line 3: Line push-ups: The students are in push-up position with their hands behind the line (outside the square). Each picks up the right hand and places it down in front of the line; then the left hand goes in front of the line. The right hand comes back behind the line, and the left hand follows. Cue with "front, front, back, back."

Line 4: Sit-ups: The students do sit-ups.

The students perform their station exercise for 30 seconds. At your signal, they jog and clap to the beat of the music as they move counterclockwise single file to the next line. Then they do the exercise for that line. Continue until the groups have completed each station twice.

60. Fitness Circuit

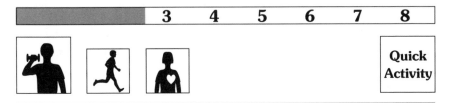

| | | 3 | 4 | 5 | 6 | 7 | 8 |

Quick Activity

Equipment: Poster of tasks

Formation: Half of class (group A) on the sidelines and endlines of the gym, half (group B) on the centerline; poster taped to the wall

2 laps jogging around gym
15 sit-ups on centerline
2 laps skipping
10 push-ups on centerline

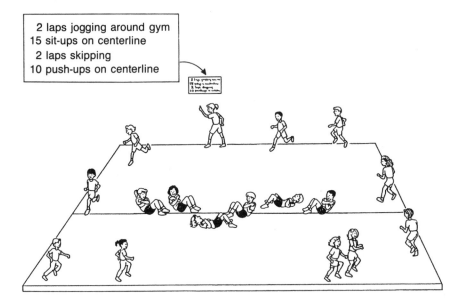

This activity allows one group to move around the gym while the other group exercises in the center. After completing a task, students begin the next task listed on the sheet. Students exercise at their own pace. They may repeat tasks once they have completed the list.

Alternate active and stationary exercises; for example, 2 laps jogging around the gym, then 10 to 15 sit-ups on the centerline; next 2 laps skipping around the gym, followed by 10 push-ups on the centerline.

61. Muscle Simon Says

		4	**5**	**6**	**7**	**8**

Quick Activity

Equipment: 4 cones, 5 jump ropes; exercise list

Formation: Personal space facing the instructor; cones section off an exercise area ("gym"); jump ropes in gym and list easily visible

This activity is played like the traditional game "Simon Says." If you begin a command with the words "Simon says," the students touch the muscle or body part you called out. If they touch a muscle without your first saying "Simon says," they must go to the "gym" and do one exercise from the list. Then they may return. Commands you may call out are limitless; for example, Simon says, touch your hamstrings; the muscle that extends your ankle; a muscle used by a ballet dancer when on tiptoe.

Exercises in the exercise area may include 10 jumping jacks, 5 push-ups, 15 sit-ups, 30 seconds of rope jumping, or 20 stomach crunches.

Variations: Allow students to be "Simon."

For an active fitness game, use commands like Simon says, jog in place; do 10 sit-ups; march; do 10 jumping jacks; take your pulse!

62. Rip City

Quick
Activity

Equipment: Waist belts with removable flags, 2 flags for each participant

Formation: Personal space

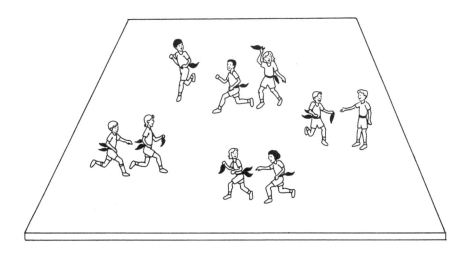

Players try to "rip" (pull) flags from the belts of other players without losing their own. Ripped flags may replace ones that have been taken by other students. If both flags are lost, that player's feet become frozen. Frozen players can get back into the game if they are able, without moving their feet, to rip a flag from someone else. Players may give flags to others who need them.

Hint: Students may not protect their flags or slap at other students. Flags must be pulled only from the belts. They may not be pulled from the hands of others.

Variations: Two teams wearing different colored flags rip flags from the opposing team while protecting their own. Players who lose both flags are out and must go to the sidelines. The team that rips all of the opposing team's flags first is the winner. This is a short activity, so students will not be out of the game for long.

For older students, incorporate soccer or basketball dribbling. Play by the same rules, but add ball handling while playing.

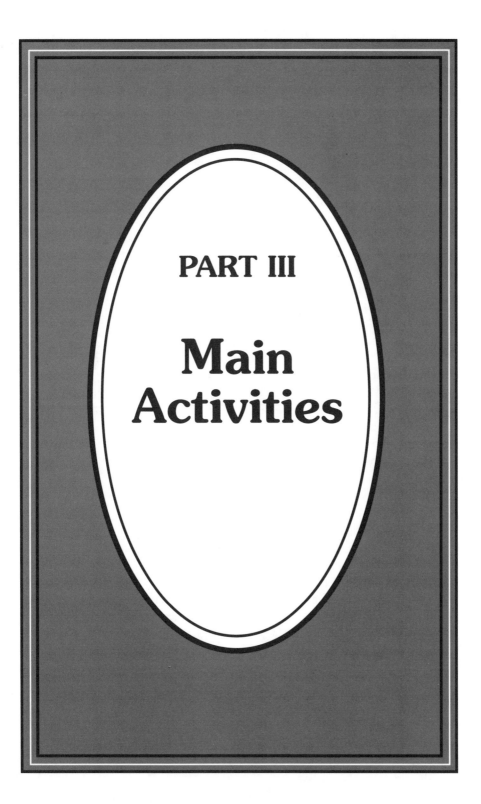

PART III

Main Activities

63. Mountain Trip

K	1	2	

Main Activity

Equipment: 1 floor hockey stick for each student

Formation: Students in single file behind instructor

Take your students on an imaginary trip, using hockey sticks to represent horses. Describe the adventure as follows: "Walk out to the corral and get your horse. What is your horse's name? Everyone, mount your horse. Are you ready to go? Let's move out slowly, single file, and follow the path (lines on the gym floor). Let's head off to the woods at a slow gallop (increase your speed). Be careful, there are low branches ahead! Bend forward and stay low. Now we are heading up the mountain. Watch out! (Slide down an imaginary mountain.) Are the horses okay? Look the horses over; check for cuts and scrapes. Everything is okay, so hop on and let's head off again. There's a water hole. Water the horses (rest time for the students). Let's take off again. This time let's gallop across the open meadow. Slow down. Walk. Now stop and tie up the horses so we can row across the river to get some food. (Sit and do a rowing motion.) Get out of the boat. Reach high and pick some apples. That's enough, we need to get going. Row back across the river. Mount the horses. Make sure they drink some water. OK, now we are heading home. Look, we are back at the corral. Everyone dismount, unsaddle your horses, and bring them into the corral."

Create a story that will keep the students moving in many ways using different pathways, levels, speeds, and locomotor and nonlocomotor movements (balancing, twisting, and bending motions). Extend the trip outside and use the features of the playground to add variety and excitement. For example, climb to the top of a slide for a mountain, use hopscotch grids as stepping-stones across a river, and use a horizontal ladder for a tunnel.

Hint: Adjust the pace carefully so that all students can keep up.

Safety Tip:

Remind students to use their hockey sticks only as horses and not to swing them or raise them into the air.

---

64. Dog Pound

K	1	2	3	

**Main
Activity**

Equipment: 1 playground or foam ball, 5-10 jump ropes per 25 students

Formation: Personal space; dog catcher in middle of playing area, a corner of which is designated the dog pound, jump ropes (dog leashes) in the pound

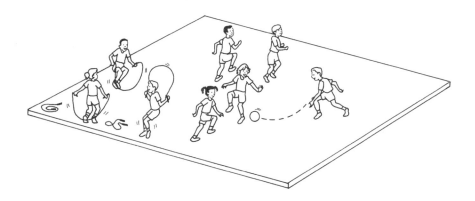

Choose one student to be the dog catcher, who calls out a locomotor movement (skip, jog, or gallop) for the other students to perform. While they are moving, the dog catcher rolls the playground ball attempting to hit someone. When students are hit, they must go to the dog pound, pick up a leash, and jump rope 10 times before returning to the game. When the dog catcher calls out "lazy dog" (at any time), all students drop to the floor and lie motionless. Any student who moves must go to the dog pound, get a leash, jump 10 times, and return to the activity. After the "lazy dog" call, the dog catcher calls out a new locomotor movement to continue the game. Change dog catchers periodically.

Variation: To get the students working at an aerobic level, let the dog catcher have several balls ready to *throw* at them. You may want to use foam balls. Select three students to retrieve balls for the dog catcher. With older students, have several dog catchers.

65. Animal Action

Main Activity

Equipment: 1 scooter for each student; 4 cones per exercise station; signs for stations

Formation: Cones at corners of exercise stations; 1 sign describing exercise at each station

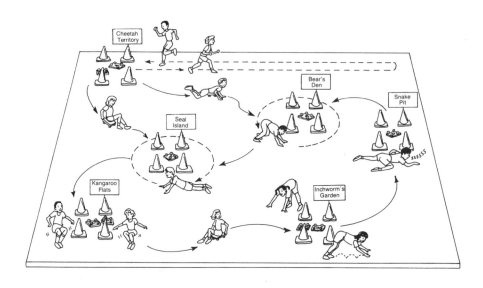

The students use scooters to travel from one station to another. They park their scooters wheels up inside the cones, perform movements characteristic of a particular animal, then move on to another station. The lines on the diagrams indicate "roads" for scooters. There are many possibilities for exercise stations.

Cheetah Territory: Students sprint down the side of the gym and back.

76

Bear's Den: Students place their hands and feet on the ground and walk, legs bent, around the outside of the den (once around the four cones).

Seal Island: Students lie on the ground and use straight arms to drag themselves around the shore of the island (once around the four cones).

Kangaroo Flats: Students jump up and down landing feet together 15 times.

Snake Pit: Students lie on their stomachs and slither like snakes around the outside of the pit (around the four cones).

Inchworm's Garden: Students place their hands and feet on the ground, walk their hands out 3 "steps" while keeping their feet stationary, then walk their feet 3 steps toward their hands. They repeat this movement 5 times.

Safety Tip:

When riding the scooters, students should keep fingers and hair away from wheels. Remember, scooters should be parked with their wheels up.

---

66. Go for Dough

Main Activity

Equipment: 4 cones; play money, assorted playground equipment (balls, scooters, jump ropes, hula hoops, basketballs, balloons, volleyballs, rackets and balls)

Formation: One cone placed near each corner of the gym; equipment off to the side

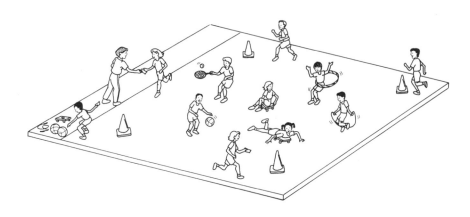

Students jog around the outside of the cones for 2 to 4 minutes depending on their ability. As they pass you, hand out play money to encourage them to jog the entire time. When the time is up, students use their play money to "buy" a piece of equipment. Each piece of "dough" will buy one item. Give them 3 to 5 minutes to exercise with the equipment and then send them jogging again to earn more money. Encourage students to buy different equipment each time, so that everyone has the chance to use each kind of equipment.

67. Health Hopping

K	1	2	3	4	5	

Equipment: For 4 stations—16 cones, 6 basketballs, 6 jump ropes, 6 mats, 6 2-ft pieces of surgical tubing; masking tape; 30 colored hula hoops

Formation: Exercise stations marked by cones; one kind of equipment and a matching exercise task at each station

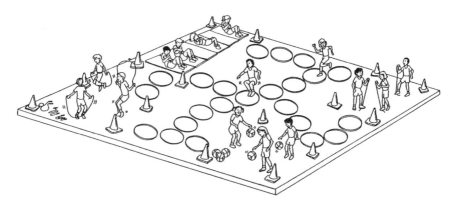

Students must travel from station to station by either jumping or hopping in and out of hoops. Be sure the hoops are securely fastened to the floor. (Flat hoops available from some equipment distributors work well for this activity.) Challenge students to travel to all of the stations and perform all the exercise tasks. Offer activities such as jumping rope 20 times, doing 10 biceps curls on each arm (step on one end of the tubing and grasp the other end), 15 bent knee sit-ups, and dribbling a basketball 15 times with each hand.

Hint: If you have enough differently colored hoops, set them up so that you make single-colored pathways to each station. Designate one color a "free" step on any color path. Then challenge students to travel to stations using one colored pathway the entire way.

Safety Tip:
Remind students *not* to snap the surgical tubing at others.

---

68. Fitness Course

K	1	2	3	4	5	6	7	8

Main Activity

Equipment: Music; miscellaneous objects (benches, mats, hurdles, hoops, ropes, gymnastic equipment, etc.)

Formation: Students move continually through the course

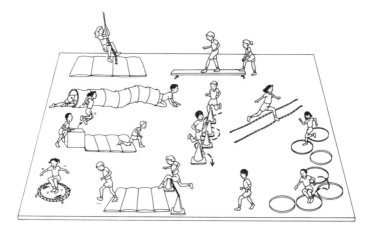

After students have completed a unit on gymnastics or jumping and landing, set up a fitness course that will keep students continually moving. Some obstacles may need to be approached from a specific direction, otherwise allow students to move freely and choose which apparatus they want to try next. Discourage lines by having the students jog to equipment where there is no wait. Though students may exercise at their own paces and skill levels, try to provide a variety of apparatus that will both accommodate them and challenge them to improve. Remember to encourage students to keep moving so their heart rates remain in their target zones.

Safety Tip:

Make sure students approach each obstacle from the appropriate direction. See that each station is properly matted.

---

69. Repeat Relays

K	1	2	3	4	5	6		

Main Activity

Equipment: None

Formation: Students paired, on opposite sides of the gym facing each other

Call out movement tasks for partners to do. For example, at your call, "High Fives," Partner A runs over to Partner B and gives a "high five," then runs back. Partner B repeats this. The variety of possible movement tasks is unlimited. You should be able to cue most using one or two words. For example, "Hand clap": A runs over and does a clapping pattern with B and runs back; B repeats.

"Crawl": A runs over, crawls through B's legs, and runs back; B repeats.

"Leap frog": A runs over to B, steps or jumps over B who is curled up in a ball, then runs back; B repeats.

"Foot clap": A runs over and sits down, facing already seated B; they both raise their feet off the ground, clap them three times, then A runs back; B repeats.

"Bump": A runs over, bumps hips gently with B, and runs back; B repeats.

70. Sharks and Surfers

| 1 | 2 | 3 | 4 | 5 |

Main Activity

Equipment: Scooters for half the class; music from "Jaws"

Formation: Two students on one side of gym, remaining students (in pairs) on the other side

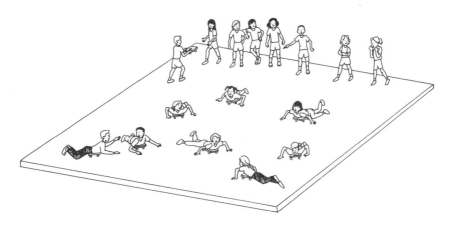

Choose two students to be sharks. The rest are surfers who lie on their surfboards (scooters) and try to paddle across the gym and back without being attacked (tagged). (The sharks are also lying on scooters.) A surfer who gets tagged on the leg or falls off the surfboard picks up the surfboard and carries it back to the sideline. The other partner then gets a turn. Partners continue to take turns as long as play continues. Stop occasionally to choose new sharks. The music adds excitement to this game!

Safety Tips:

Have students practice pulling and pushing themselves on the scooters, remembering to keep their fingers away from scooter wheels. Tie back long hair so it does not get tangled in the wheels.

---

71. Movement Fun

Main Activity

Equipment: Hoops, ribbons, scarves, towels; music

Formation: Personal space

The objective of this activity is to maintain a target heart rate while moving continually. Teach students movements to do with the different kinds of equipment. If you are using scarves, move them in different levels, move them at different speeds, make different shapes, and write names in the air. Have students try combinations of these movements while performing a specific routine. Then give them the opportunity to move to music throughout the gym. Move with the children—this gives them the encouragement and the confidence to move freely. Choose a second piece of equipment and lead another small series of movements. Let the students create and explore movements by themselves. Repeat this pattern using each kind of equipment. Exploring movement with equipment keeps students interested while they create a fun aerobic workout! Remind students to keep their heart rates within their target zones.

72. Crab Soccer

| 1 | 2 | 3 | 4 | 5 |

Equipment: 5 soccer balls

Formation: Half of class in personal space in crabwalk position; half in short lines

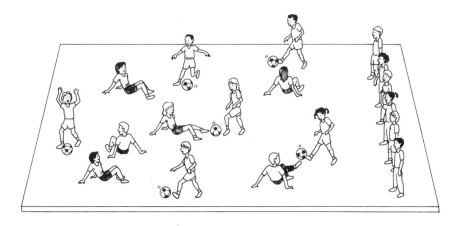

The first person in each line attempts to dribble the ball from one sideline to the other through the field of crabs. The crabs try to touch a ball with one foot while crabwalking. A crab who touches a ball switches places with the dribbler. The students who are crabs must stay in the crabwalk position. They cannot turn over and crawl or get up and walk. Dribblers must keep their balls close to themselves and maintain ball control using feet only. After a while, have the first group of crabs become dribblers and the dribblers become crabs.

Variation: For a closing activity, have three students take the crab position and the remaining students each take a ball. This time, the crabs try to tag the *students* as they dribble around on the playing field. Tagged players put their balls away and become crabs. Continue until all the players have become crabs. This is a great way to collect balls at the end of class.

73. Hideout

Main Activity

Equipment: 4 "hideouts" (folding mats or big cardboard boxes); foam balls for half the class; tape or cones

Formation: 1 hideout at each corner of the gym; 4 or 5 students in the center of gym (throwers) and the rest behind hideouts (runners)

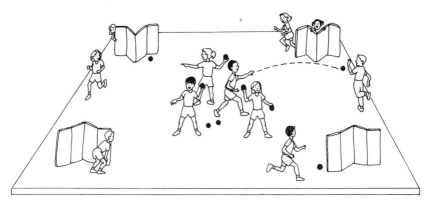

The runners try to move from one hideout to the next without being hit by balls. They may duck behind the hideouts as they run, but only for 5 seconds, and then they must move on to the next one. The throwers may start counting—1, 2, 3, 4, 5—to get the runners moving. Once a runner leaves a hideout he or she must go to the next one. Any runner hit by a ball is out and goes to the sidelines. The throwers must stay inside the throwing area marked off with tape, cones, or painted gym lines. Two of the throwers are retrievers; they go after balls and either throw or roll them back to the throwing area. Runners and throwers trade places when all the runners are out or after 2 minutes of play.

Safety Tip:

Establish one-way for running for safety. Remind runners that once they start running, they may not go back to the last hideout.

---

74. Double-Double

**Main
Activity**

Equipment: 1 marker per student; chalk

Formation: 3-4 students at each jumping game

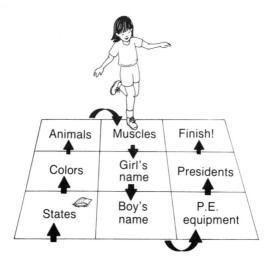

Animals	Muscles	Finish!
Colors	Girl's name	Presidents
States	Boy's name	P.E. equipment

This game is played similarly to hopscotch on a grid drawn on the playground. The objective is to move a marker through the squares by progressing through each category.

Players start in the lower left hand corner of the grid. Each begins by tossing a marker into the square labeled States, then hops on one foot two times in that square while calling out "States, States."

The player proceeds through the grid by calling out a different state twice while hopping two times in each square; for example: First square, "States, States"; second square, "Maine, Maine"; third square, "Oregon, Oregon"; etc. A student who successfully hops through the entire grid tosses the marker to the next square, Colors. This continues until the student steps on a line, makes a mistake calling out a name, is unable to think of a name for a particular category, or misses the square when tossing the marker. The student then forfeits his or her turn and the next person begins.

Hint: Allow younger students to use some of the lines as stepping-stones to help them reach the squares they are starting in.

Variation: Numerous categories may be used in place of those shown; for example, birds, insects, trees, cars, food. For a shorter game, draw a grid of 6 squares instead of 9.

75. Fit Stop

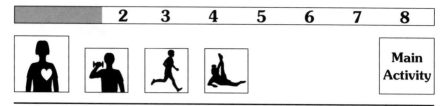

	2	3	4	5	6	7	8

Main Activity

Equipment: 5-8 jump ropes, 5-8 pieces of surgical tubing 4 feet long, 6-10 cones, 1-2 basketballs; exercise signs; music

Formation: Partners equally positioned at different exercise stations (fit stops); an exercise instruction sheet and appropriate equipment at each fit stop; cones at each corner of the gym

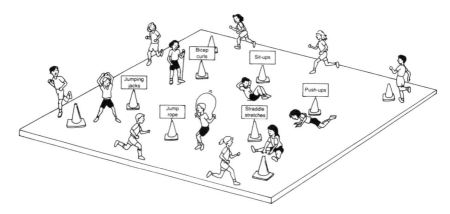

After you explain all of the fit stops to the class, have one partner of each pair pick a station to begin at. The other partner begins jogging around the cones while the fit-stopper does the prescribed exercise for the length of time it takes the jogger to complete 1 lap. They then trade places; the jogger begins working at the fit stop and the fit-stopper jogs 1 lap. When the second jogger finishes the lap, the partners rotate to another fit-stop. You can create a variety of innovative fit stops by using available equipment and your imagination.

Fit stops may include straddle stretches (see p. 22), stomach crunches, bent knee sit-ups, push-ups, rope jumping, strength exercises (such as biceps curls, or triceps extensions using tubing), or aerobic movements (such as mountain climbers, skiers, jumping jacks, and grapevine steps).

76. We Stretch, They Stretch

K	1	2	3		

Main Activity

Equipment: Music

Formation: Personal space

Discuss how different things bend and stretch: weeping willow tree, robot, bird, sunflower, snake, ballet dancer, a person throwing a ball, someone reaching up high. When the music begins, call out a locomotor movement for the students to do until the music stops. Then tell them to stretch like a tree (for example) until the music begins again. When the music starts, call out another locomotor movement. Students stop stretching and begin traveling again. Ideas for traveling movements include skip, hop, jog, racewalk, bearwalk, gallop, slide, skip and turn, jump turn, grapevine, polka, and any combination of these. Or let students choose their own locomotor movements. They will think of wonderful and creative ways to stretch too!

77. Guard Your Pin

Main Activity

Equipment: 1 pin and 1 fleece ball for every student ("pins" can be plastic bowling pins, wooden pins, carpet tubes, or milk cartons)

Formation: Pins scattered on gym floor; students guard their own pins

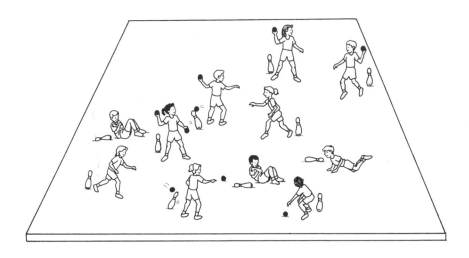

Students throw balls at each other's standing pins while guarding their own pins. When a pin is knocked down, that student performs an exercise that will develop muscular strength, such as sit-ups, push-ups, line jumps, and wall push-ups. Students return to the game when they complete their exercises.

Variations:

Soccer: Students kick balls to knock down pins and use their feet to trap the ball.

Hockey: Students use a hockey stick to control a puck with which they knock pins down; they may guard their own pins with their hockey sticks or their feet.

Partners: Partners may play any of the previous games; one plays the defensive position and the other plays the offensive position.

Teams: Divide the gym between two teams. Play until all the pins on one side are down. The team with pins still standing does 5 sit-ups and the other team does 10 sit-ups.

78. Hoop Out

**Main
Activity**

Equipment: 3 bases, 2 hula hoops, 1 bat, 1 ball

Formation: Students divided into 2 teams, one outfield, the other at bat

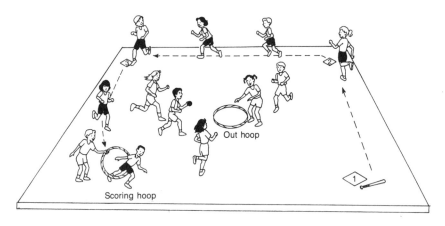

In this game, the *whole team* "runs the bases" when their batter hits the ball. The running pathway consists of three bases and one hoop. A player from the fielding team holds the hoop up for the runners to go through. Each runner who completes a circuit of the pathway scores 1 run. Runners must stop when the ball has been retrieved and placed in the "out" hoop and *each* fielder has a hand or foot inside the out hoop.

You may let five batters hit before changing sides, or an entire team may bat before the other team hits. You are the pitcher. There are no strike outs.

Hints: You may want to offer batters a choice of a pitch or a batting tee. Use a larger, softer ball for younger players. A baseball diamond can be used for the runners' pathway.

Variation: This game may be played with kicking skills instead of batting skills.

79. Scooter-Chute

	4	5	6	

**Main
Activity**

Equipment: Parachute; scooters for half the students

Formation: Students in pairs around parachute, one holding the parachute, the other on a scooter

There are many activities you may have the students perform. The following are examples.

Parachute-partners hold on to the chute with one hand and hold their partners one hand with the other. The scooter-partners sit on the scooters and hold on with their free hands. The parachute-partners walk clockwise with the chute while pulling their partners. On your signal, the students stop and reverse directions.

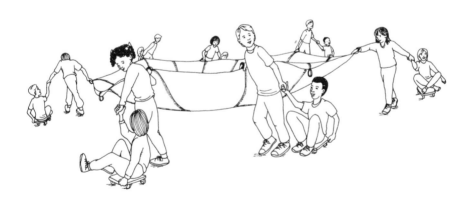

Parachute-partners hold on to the chute with both hands. Scooter-partners lie on their stomachs facing the center of the chute. As the parachute-partners raise the chute up into a "cloud," the scooter-partners go under the chute to the center, meet other scooters, and retreat backwards before the cloud collapses.

93

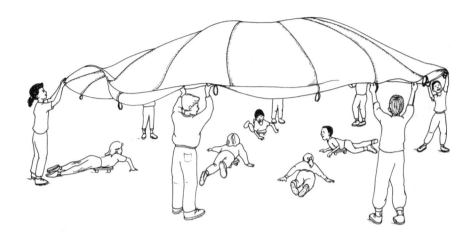

Parachute-partners make waves with the parachute by holding it at waist-level and moving it up and down in a rapid motion. Scooter-partners on their stomachs move in a circle under the chute.

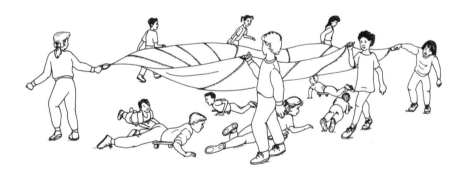

Parachute-partners make a mountain by lifting the parachute high above their heads, pulling it rapidly down to the ground, and kneeling on the edge of the chute to trap the air inside. The scooter-partners travel around the mountain either clockwise or counterclockwise. Or, when the chute is lifted up, the scooters move underneath it and remain stationary while the mountain stands.

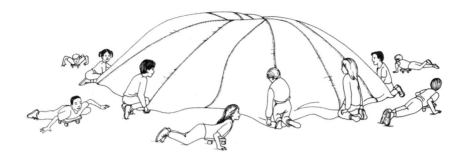

This final maneuver takes some precision: As parachute-partners lift the chute to form a cloud, scooter-partners, sitting on the scooters, move quickly into the center. When the parachute has reached its peak, the parachute-partners walk in 4 steps and the chute rises higher into a mushroom shape. The scooter-partners move out as the parachute-partners move in.

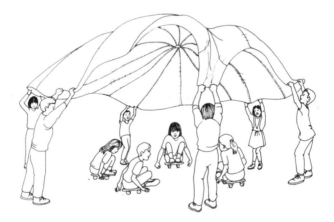

Let partners trade places and try the maneuvers again. Have students create other group movements after they have worked together a while.

Safety Tips:
Remind students to keep their fingers clear of the scooter wheels and long hair tucked back. The students holding the parachute need to be aware of where the students on scooters are as they manipulate the chute.

80. Skipper's Delight

		4	5	6	7	8

Main Activity

Equipment: 6-8 long jump ropes

Formation: Long jump ropes set up as shown in diagram, several students lined up behind each rope

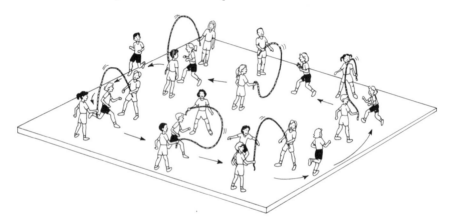

This is a continuous activity that lets students practice entering and exiting a long rope. The students move around the gym running through each rope they come to. All of the ropes are turned "front-doors" (i.e., toward the jumpers), so students can move from one rope to another without stopping. Students do not need to wait for a turn. They should continue moving even if several students run through at the same time. Allow students who are turning the ropes to exchange places with the students running through after a set period.

After all can move through the course doing front-doors, have students practice with the rope turning "back-doors" (i.e., away from the jumpers). When doing back-doors, students must jump the rope at least once before running out. Challenge students by mixing the directions the ropes are turned, by having them reverse the direction in which they travel from rope to rope at your signal, or by having them try to go through while holding hands with their partners.

81. Wacky-Ball

	4	5	6	7	8

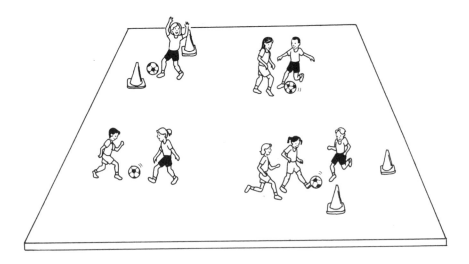

Main Activity

Equipment: 4 foam soccer balls, 4 cones for goals

Formation: 2 teams, 1 on each side of gym

This is a continuous indoor soccer game designed to improve basic soccer skills and to allow more opportunities for players to make contact with a ball. Emphasize keeping the ball low and using fundamental soccer skills such as controlled dribbling and passing to a partner while moving the ball down the field. Players may not touch the ball with their hands. When a goal is scored, the ball is kicked back into the flow of the game. There are no out-of-bounds when playing in an enclosed area such as a gym. Outside you may designate a boundary line.

82. All-Star Action

	4	5	6	7	8

Main
Activity

Equipment: 5-10 basketballs (or foam basketballs); 4 bases

Formation: Bases set up like a baseball field on one half of the gym, a basketball court on the other end; 2 teams, 1 at the basketball court positioned around the hoop, the other standing single file at home plate

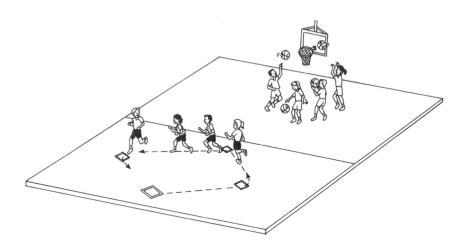

On your signal, the team at the basket begins shooting and keeping count of the number of baskets they make. At the same time, the other team runs the bases as quickly as they can, all together in single file. The last runner to cross home plate calls out "Stop," and the other team stops shooting. The teams switch sides and repeat this activity for a predetermined number of "innings." The team that scores the most *baskets*, wins.

83. Fitness Freedom

| | | 4 | 5 | 6 | 7 | 8 | |

Main Activity

Equipment: 5 jump ropes, 5 hoops, 5 basketballs, 5 playground balls, 5 pieces of surgical tubing; chalkboard, chalk

Formation: Personal space; equipment on the floor around the gym

This activity challenges students to exercise continuously for 15 to 20 minutes while using a variety of equipment. For example, a student may jump rope for 5 minutes, shoot basketballs for 5 minutes, then twirl a hoop, bounce a ball against a wall, or practice aerobic movements, such as galloping, skipping, hopping, grapevine, or sliding, for the last 5 minutes. Challenge students to use their imaginations. (Their creativity can be limitless. You may learn some new ideas!)

At regular intervals (e.g., every 2 minutes), single out a student who is working well and write his or her name on the chalkboard in large letters. At each interval, when a new person is selected, write the previous name to one side of the chalkboard and the newcomer's name in large letters. When the class is over, read the entire list aloud.

Hint: Fitness Freedom is best played after students have been involved in a unit of fitness instruction. Ideas you presented then may be applied by the students in this activity.

84. Water-Skiing

Main Activity

Equipment: Carpet square and 1 rope for every 2 students

Formation: Students in pairs at one end of gym

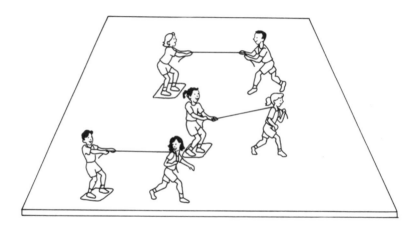

One partner "water-skis" using the inverted carpet square like a ski and holding one end of the rope. The other partner is the "boat" and holds the other end of the rope. The two partners work together to travel down the gym, the skier first sitting, then kneeling, and finally standing. The boat must pull strongly enough to counterbalance the skier in the standing position. Finding the balancing position is critical to the skier's success. With practice and a strong, steady boat, students will learn how to maintain the best balance. Have the partners switch roles each time they reach the end of the gym.

Safety Tip:

Students should move up and down the gym *or* in the same direction around a large circle. Remind students not to jerk the ropes, but to pull at a steady rate and to go the speed their skiers are comfortable with.

---

85. Strength Challenge

	4	**5**	**6**	**7**	**8**

Main Activity

Equipment: Climbing rope; chin-up bar; several mats; 2 stopwatches; masking tape; 1 scoresheet and pencil for each student

Formation: 1 station for each of the following: sit-ups, push-ups, pull-ups, rope climb, vertical jump, standing broad jump

Students are to go to every station and accumulate as many points as possible. Explain each station and its scoring, then give each student a Strength Challenge scoresheet that you have designed.

Push-Ups: Each push-up completed earns 1 point. Students have 1 minute to do push-ups. Students time each other.

Sit-Ups: Every third repetition earns 1 point. Students have 1 minute to do sit-ups, sitting on a mat, hands placed across the chest; a partner may hold their feet. Students time each other.

Pull-Ups: Each repetition earns 2 points. Arms should be fully extended on the down phase of the pull-up. There is no time limit.

Vertical Jump: On a strip of tape stuck to the wall, mark off a baseline (e.g., 4 ft. above the floor) and each inch above that to 6-8 ft (higher if students are able). From a standing position, students jump up and touch the tape. The number of inches touched *above* the baseline equals the number of points earned.

Standing Broad Jump: Mark off sections on a strip of tape stuck on a mat to designate points earned. From a standing position students push off with both feet. The longer the jump, the greater the number of points earned.

Rope Climb: Section the rope into thirds with pieces of tape. Each section climbed is worth 1 point; climb 2 sections, earn 2 points. A student who touches the ceiling earns 4 points.

Safety Tip:

Make sure the rope climb and the standing broad jump are properly matted.
